Haircutting Basics

*An easy, step-by-step guide
to cutting hair the professional way.*

Martha G. Fernandez

Illustrated by
Dacil Hernandez

Revised, Expanded 1991 Edition

Good Life Products, Inc.
P.O. Box 170070
Hialeah, FL 33017-0070

(305) 362-6998

Haircutting Basics

*An easy, step-by-step guide
to cutting hair the professional way.*

Martha G. Fernandez

Illustrated by
Dacil Hernandez

Published by

Good Life Products, Inc.
Post Office Box 170070
Hialeah, FL 33017-0070 U.S.A.

First Printing, 1988
Second Printing, 1989
Revised, Expanded Edition, 1991

Library of Congress Cataloging-in-Publication Data.

Fernandez, Martha G.,   1954-
   Haircutting basics   :   an easy, step-by-step guide to cutting hair
the professional way / Martha G. Fernandez ;   illustrated by Dacil
Hernandez. -- Rev., expanded 1991 ed.
      p.   cm.
   Includes bibliographical references and index
   ISBN 0-944460-21-6   : $16.95
   1. Haircutting.   I. Title.
TT970. F47 1991
646.7' 242--dc20   90-22006
                                                                CIP

DISCLAIMER

Anyone who wishes to cut hair with accuracy must expect to dedicate time to practice and gain expertise.

The purpose of this book is to inform, educate, and entertain its readers. The author and *Good Life Products, Inc.* shall have neither liability or responsibility to any person or entity with respect to any loss or damage caused or alleged to be caused directly or indirectly by the information contained in this book.

ATTENTION SCHOOLS

This book is available at special quantity discount,
for details write to:

Good Life Products, Inc.
Special Sales Dept.
P.O. Box 170070
Hialeah, FL 33017-0070

(305) 362-6998

TABLE OF CONTENTS

ACKNOWLEDGMENTS

I would like to thank Margarita Zepeda for the skillful drawings she added to the new chapter, and Jim Cheetham for his criticism. I owe a special thank you to Maria V. Vila, who went to such trouble to review my manuscript and who made so many helpful suggestions and corrections, although of course I remain entirely responsible for any mistakes the book may still contain. I am also deeply appreciative to my husband, who offered his patient labor to put the final touches into the book. Finally I would like to thank all the students who have called or written, to tell me how this humble book has contributed to their success.

M.G.F.

INTRODUCTION

Haircutting is the art of changing the hair into a style, mainly to provide a more attractive and neat appearance. The art of cutting hair has been practiced in a variety of cultures since ancient times when hairdressing demanded processing and adornment. Today, there are techniques for wash-and-wear haircuts that may be styled in a conservative or sophisticated fashion to express the individual's character.

Because there are so many different ways to cut hair and a wide range of hairstyles, today's student needs an easy step-by-step method to cut hair quickly and efficiently. This book was designed for beginners who are in the process of training to become future haircutters; for the graduates of beauty school who haven't mastered a technique of their own; and for those interested in learning a simple haircutting technique to take care of their friends' and families' hairstyling needs.

Among the goals of this book is to keep technical jargon to a minimum and to provide an easy-to-follow format for the beginner. The material is therefore organized from the basic and essential information to complex training. Furthermore, this new edition includes some of the latest clipper cutting techniques to prepare the individual for more advanced hairstyles.

Many people are afraid to cut hair because they think cutting is too complicated, in fact haircutting is like any other skill such as typewriting or playing the guitar, which requires regular practice to be mastered well. Once the student has learned and practiced these methods, the fundamental techniques of haircutting will provide the foundation to learn advanced methods of creating different hairstyles and effects.

This book presents a standard technique that is simple, effective, and easy to learn. By repeating the step-by-step methods described, the student will quickly develop speed and accuracy. A Glossary, Index, and numerous illustrations are included to help any beginning haircutter, whether young or old, student or professional. With that thought in mind, the book provides a unique and precise method of instruction. Through constant practice and study, the beginning student will develop the experience necessary to master basic haircutting.

For best results, this book should first be read thoroughly for an overview of the subject. Then, the actual hands-on practice begins. Ask a friend who has confidence in you to let you practice the haircutting technique. Choose a particular hairstyle, place the book on a table and follow the steps indicated. The type is large enough to be read at a distance.

Once you have practiced the various haircutting methods, your confidence, and, therefore, your speed and accuracy, should grow. After mastering the basics of proper haircutting, you can move on to more sophisticated techniques and develop your own style and specialty. For now, however, your challenge is to learn the basics described here in simple terms for the benefit of the at-home amateur or the student. Good luck!

M.G.F.

Chapter I

FUNDAMENTALS

There are many variables to a good haircut--the tools, the type and condition of the hair, the technique employed, and the facial characteristics and physique of the individual. To obtain successful haircuts you need to have knowledge of these variables; they're the fundament to understand why the hair behaves as it does and what results will be obtained when you give a haircut.

In this Chapter you will learn about those variables to prepare you for Chapter II--haircutting technique in depth.

A. THE TOOLS

The Scissors

There are a wide range of haircutting scissors in the market. Once you have spent some time cutting hair with different types of scissors, you will be able to determine which one suits you best. In precision haircutting the hair is cut with the tips of the scissors; this is why it is recommended to use the mini-scissors. Their small size, from four to five and a half inches, fits the hand comfortably and the short blades give better control when cutting sides and corners. *Fig. 1.1.*

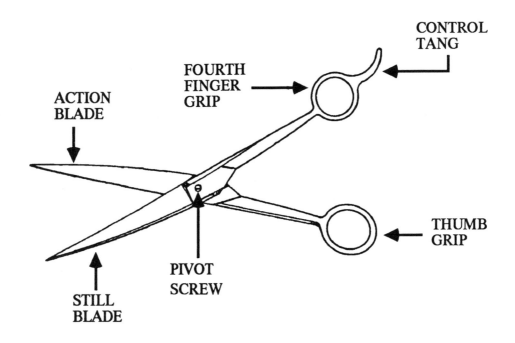

Fig 1.1

Usually long blade scissors are used in barber styling techniques in combination with the comb where the lengths to cut are long across the head. To cut the layers with uniformity using this technique, long blade scissors are necessary. Small scissors would cut small sections and the layers would be uneven.

The control tang is not necessary, but try it; it may help you maintain the scissors in balance while you cut.

Prices for scissors range from a few dollars to over a hundred. You'll have to determine which one is affordable to you. It is not necessary to invest in an expensive pair of scissors, but those with low quality will cut unevenly. There is a wide selection of scissors made in Solingen, West Germany. Solingen is a city famous for its steel and iron ware; the scissors made there are exported to all parts of the world. The ice-tempered stainless is good and reasonably priced. Check the Appendix for information on how to obtain good quality scissors.

The blades should be dried after each haircut, and residues of hair should be cleaned. The pivot screw and the inside of the blades should be kept clean and oiled with clipper type oil. When needed, the blades of your fine shears should be sharpened by a sharpening and honing expert. They know what the needs of different types of scissors are for optimum sharpness and edge holding durability. I've had scissors ruined by grinders that have completely removed the teeth or broken the blades. So be smarter than I was; ask for a guaranteed job.

Be careful with your scissors. If you drop them the points may be damaged and they may lose their pivot screw adjustment.

The pivot screw should not be too tight or loose. To find out if it is properly adjusted, hold the scissors horizontally by the thumb grip (pivot screw facing you,) open wide the upper grip and let it drop. If the tips of the scissors are more than one-eight of an inch open, the screw is too tight; if the tips are closed, the screw is too loose. The tips of the scissors should stop at a distance of one-eight of an inch from each other when the still blade drops. Proper adjustment will prevent damage to the hair and to the scissors. *Fig. 1.2.*

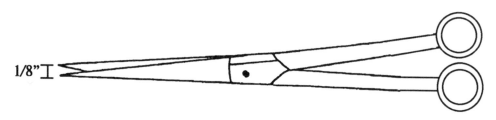

PROPERLY ADJUSTED SCISSORS

Fig. 1.2

Thinning Shears

Thinning shears are used to reduce hair bulk. There are two types of thinning shears.

a) <u>Notched Single Edge Scissor</u> *Fig. 1.3.*

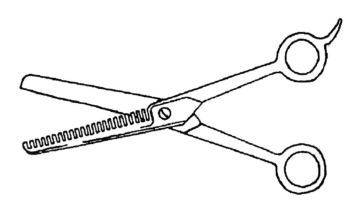

Fig. 1.3

b) <u>Notched Double Edge Scissor</u>

Shears with teeth on one blade take off more hair than those with teeth on both blades. *Fig. 1.4.*

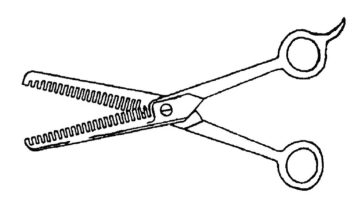

Fig. 1.4

These are some general rules to thin out the hair correctly with thinning shears:

1) Thinning is done in the underlying layers of the hair; the top layers should be longer to cover the hair that has been thinned out.

2) Don't thin out too much hair.

3) Don't thin hairline hair.

4) Don't thin the hair too close to the scalp. Start thinning the hair at least one inch away from the scalp.

5) Thin the hair in small even sections.

6) Place the scissors in a vertical or a diagonal direction to avoid steps in the hair. Straight hair will show a chopped look.

7) Work your way from the top to the bottom in spaced intervals.

8) Don't close the scissors partially. It will give more damage to the hair.

9) Don't thin the hair before a permanent wave. You need even sections of hair to roll it easily on the rods.

A precision haircut cannot be accomplished if it involves thinning the hair. The reason is that thinning gives the hair uneven lengths. To thin the hair correctly, the techniques must be practiced, otherwise you can spoil a good haircut. I prefer to use the thinning shears to create special effects, or to give volume to some areas of the hairstyle. You will learn some of these techniques in Chapter III.

The razor, *Fig. 1.5,* may also be used to thin out the hair. Razor cutting and thinning sharpens the ends of the hair, scratches the cortex, and creates split and dry, fly away ends.

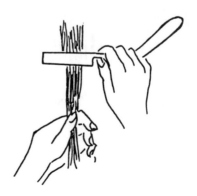

THE RAZOR

Fig. 1.5

Slithering is another method to thin the hair. The scissors are slidden up and down the underside of a strand of hair; they are closed slightly on each stroke toward the head, then opened as they are brought back. This method can scratch and partially cut the cortex.

Many people note that when their hair was thinned out it became unmanageable after a couple of weeks. The shorter ends, as they grew, pushed the longer hair making it seem even bulkier. People with coarse, curly, and of thick density hair often want it thinned out. Usually these types of hair tend to push more as they grow. So, unless you plan to give an exotic style that requires thinning, it is best to shape the hair with a precision haircut--it will last longer and with the right haircut you can diminish bulk.

The Comb

The hair will be handled better with a hard, sturdy comb. One half should have the teeth set wide apart; the other fine closed set teeth. The wide teeth are used to untangle hair. To untangle hair start at the ends and work your way up to the top, half an inch at a time. The fine teeth are used to smooth the hair once it has been untangled. Either side can be used to lift the hair. You may want to use the wide teeth to lift thick hair, and the closed set teeth to lift fine hair. *Fig. 1.6.* Combs that lose their teeth should be discarded, they cause damage and comb the hair unevenly.

BACK

WIDE TEETH   FINE TEETH

Fig. 1.6

B. THE HAIR

Hair Structure

Hair is mostly protein. When observed under a microscope you can see that the hair has three layers *(fig. 1.7.)* The cuticle is the outer layer composed of tiny overlapping scales made of hard protein. This hard protein is called keratin; it protects the hair and holds moisture.

The hair looks dull and dry when the cuticle is open or broken. Some of this damage occurs if the hair is over-processed with chemicals, burned by a hot drier applied too close to the hair, over-exposure to the sun or chlorine, and even by brushing it and pulling it when wet. Alkaline products applied to the hair will open the cuticle and make it sensitive to breakage.

pH balanced shampoos and conditioners are recommended to close the cuticle's scales, and make the hair feel soft and look shiny.

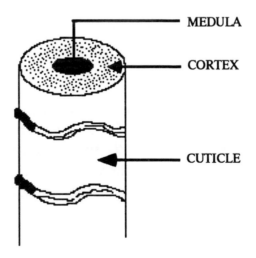

MEDULA

CORTEX

CUTICLE

HAIR STRUCTURE

Fig. 1.7

The cortex is the layer next to the cuticle. This is where melanin, the pigment that gives the hair color, is produced. The medulla is the innermost layer of cells in the hair. It is not known what is the purpose of the medulla. *Fig. 1.7.*

Form, Texture, and Density of Hair

Each hair grows out of a tiny tube in the scalp called the follicle. In its base the papilla produces the cells necessary for hair growth and it nourishes the follicle with blood and oxygen. If the papilla is damaged or destroyed, it will not produce hair. *Fig. 1.8.*

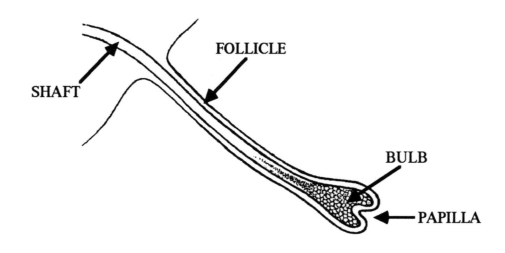

PARTS OF THE ROOT

Fig. 1.8

There are four major forms of hair: 1) straight, 2) wavy, 3) curly, and 4) super-curly. The shape of the hair follicle determines the form that the hair will have. Detailed in figure 1.9 are the different relationships between the shape of the hair follicle and the forms of hair that will result. Each of these forms can be fine, medium or coarse in texture. The texture is determined by the size of the cortex that makes the hair shaft thicker or thinner. Fine textured hair is soft and shiny; it tends to go limp, flat, and won't hold a set. Medium textured hair has body and bounce; it has a strong direction, so it's better to style it following its own natural pattern. The ends may feel coarse, dry, and prone to split ends. With rich conditioners the hair may go limp. Coarse hair lacks shine. It is dry, bulky, wiry, and it requires extra care such as rich conditioners, the right cut, and styling aids to control its bulk.

Hair density refers to the amount of strands per square inch. Blonds have the most density, brown and black haired follow, and red heads have the least density. Rather than dealing with the number of hairs per square inch we will define density as thin, medium or thick. To determine the density of a specific head of hair look for these clues: Is the scalp visible when the hair is wet or dry? Do conditioners make the hair flat? Is the hair bushy? Does it need gel or other styling aids to control it? The density is thin if the scalp shows through the hair and conditioners flatten the hair. The density is medium if the scalp does not show when the hair is wet or dry and it does not appear bushy, and it is thick if the hair has lots of bulk and styling aids are needed to control it.

Usually curly and super-curly hair (because they coil out from the scalp,) as well as any hair that is coarse, tend to be bulky. Super-curly hair is specially fragile because is has a thin cortex, and it is usually processed with strong harsh chemicals that make it dry and prone to breakage. These types of hair will look more attractive with a layered cut to shape the hair, reduce its volume, and eliminate the split ends. On the other side, fine hair, also with a thin cortex, will appear thicker with a blunt cut. *Fig. 1.9.*

FORMS OF HAIR

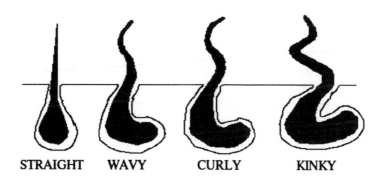

STRAIGHT WAVY CURLY KINKY

Shape of The Follicle	Forms of Hair
round	straight hair
oval	wavy hair
almost flat	curly hair
flat	super-curly hair

Fig. 1.9

21

Growth of Hair

Hair length is the distance between the base of the hair to the end of the hair. *Fig. 1.10.*

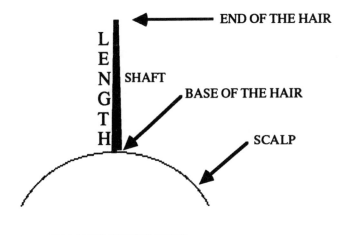

GROWTH OF THE HAIR

Fig 1.10

The hair shaft grows about half an inch per month. For short hair you can recommend monthly trims because uneven lengths show sooner than in long hair. Long hair can wait six to eight weeks to be trimmed.

Healthy dry hair stretches up to one-fifth of its normal length when held tautly, springing back to its original length when released. Wet with water it will stretch almost half its length. Therefore, when you cut it wet and stretched it will be shorter after it dries. *Fig. 1.11.*

Special care should be taken when cutting hair with body, coarse or curly. After the hair dries and curls it will be shorter than a straight form of hair.

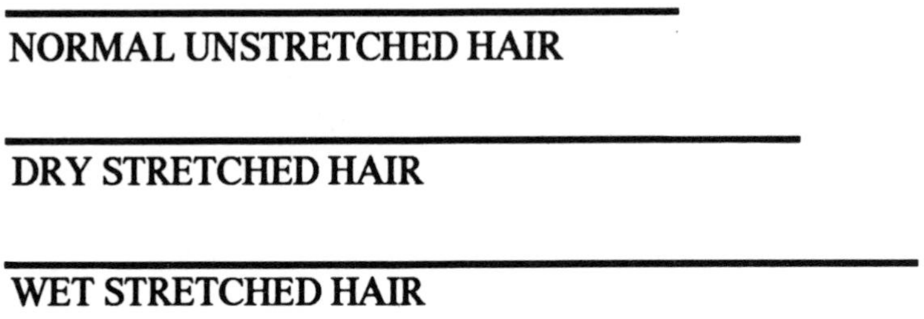

NORMAL UNSTRETCHED HAIR

DRY STRETCHED HAIR

WET STRETCHED HAIR

Fig. 1.11

All hair go through a process of three different phases called Anagen, Catagen, and Telogen. The papilla controls these phases. Anagen is the growing phase; most of the hair is in this phase which lasts two to six years. After the Anagen, there is a resting period called Catagen during which the follicle is dormant. At the end of the cycle comes the Telogen phase. In this phase the hair falls each day in a shedding process, replacing the old hair with new. Age, failing health, trauma, pregnancy, drugs, poor diet, and constantly pulling the hair with pony tails may cause temporary baldness or slow hair growth.

Many people believe that shaving the children's hair will stimulate the growth of strong, abundant hair. Shaving will not change the kind of hair a person has. The genes determine the papilla and follicle located in the interior layers of the scalp and it will not change by shaving the hair shaft. As the child grows the hair will go through several stages, it may become stronger and thicker, or remain fine.

C. EXERCISES

The following exercises have been designed to help you accomplish the objectives listed below. Practice them carefully to be able to learn the haircutting technique explained in this book. Once you become proficient in your practice of these exercises, you can move on to the next section. If you have had some instruction and are familiar with these objectives, go on to more complex material.

Objectives:

1) To be able to hold the scissors correctly.
2) To be able to hold the scissors and the comb correctly.
3) To be able to hold the scissors and the comb correctly while combing the hair.
4) To be able to hold and move the scissors, the comb, and the hair correctly while cutting.
5) To develop speed while manipulating the tools and the hair.

Note that the dominant hand (meaning your right if you are right handed, or your left if you are left handed) manipulates the scissors and combs the hair. The opposite hand holds the hair to be cut, determines how much hair will be cut, and holds the comb while the dominant hand is cutting.

Exercise #1. Hold the scissors with your dominant hand. Face the scissors' pivot screw toward your chest. Insert the thumb in the thumb grip and the ring finger in the fourth finger grip. If your scissors have control tang rest your little finger on it. Fingers should be inserted up to the first joint. Once you have the correct hand position, open and close the scissors only moving the action blade. Your thumb will be doing the work, while the still blade, controlled by the ring finger, remains motionless.

Action: Open, close. Repeat increasing speed. *Fig. 1.12.*

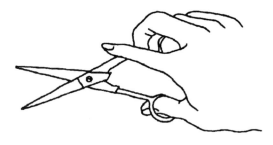

Fig. 1.12

Exercise #2. Hold the scissors as practiced. Close the blades; and keeping the ring finger inside the fourth finger grip, remove the thumb from its grip and hold the scissors in the palm of your hand. Now, insert the thumb back into its grip and open and close the scissors three times as learned in the previous exercise. Repeat the entire exercise twenty times trying to increase speed.

Action: Remove the thumb, hold scissors in palm, insert the thumb, open and close scissors. Repeat increasing speed. *Fig. 1.13-1.14.*

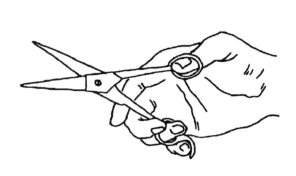

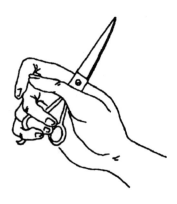

Fig. 1.13   *Fig. 1.14*

Exercise #3. With scissors in the palm of your hand, take hold of the back of the comb with your index finger and thumb of the same hand. In this position, comb the hair of a friend or a wig lifting the hair up and letting it drop. Repeat ten times. Start on the left side of the head and move towards the right. (Beware of the tips of the scissors. In this position someone could be accidentally hurt.)

Action: Hold closed scissors and comb the hair up, drop hair. Repeat increasing speed. *Fig. 1.15.*

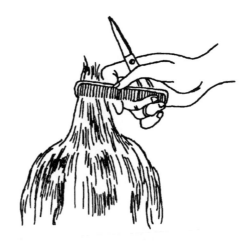

Fig 1.15

Exercise #4. With scissors and comb in the palm of your dominant hand, comb the hair up and hold it between the middle and index fingers of your opposite hand. Drop the hair, and repeat the procedure five times moving from left to right.

Action: Hold closed scissors and comb, comb hair up, hold hair with fingers, drop hair. Repeat. *Fig. 1.16.*

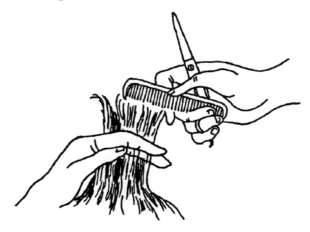

Fig. 1.16

25

Exercise #5. Repeat exercise four, but do not drop the hair. Instead, transfer the comb to the opposite hand and hold the teeth in the curb of your hand, using the thumb to secure it in place. Insert the thumb in the scissors' grip and pretend cutting. Remove the thumb from its grip and hold the scissors in the palm of your hand. Return the comb to the dominant hand. Drop the hair. Repeat the exercise combing the hair from left to right, transferring the comb back and forth, trying to gain speed.

Action: Hold comb and closed scissors with dominant hand (ring finger in its grip), comb hair up, hold hair with fingers, transfer comb, insert thumb in its grip, pretend cutting, hold closed scissors in palm, transfer comb back to dominant hand, and drop hair. Repeat. *Fig. 1.17.*

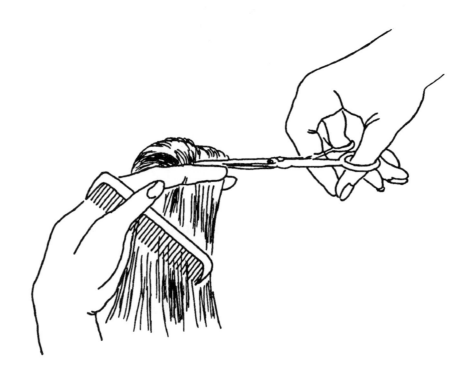

Fig. 1.17

Now you have had an introduction to how to handle the tools and the hair. Later while giving the practice haircuts explained in Chapter II, you will gain control and speed. Remember that the more you practice these exercises the better prepared you will be to cut hair. The goal is to handle the tools in an automatic way so you can fully concentrate on the cutting technique.

D. LEARN YOUR ANGLES

In the course of this book you will give several practice haircuts; some of the haircuts will be layered.

Layers are progressive graduations of the hair, from short to long, or from long to short. In order to cut layers, small sections of hair are elevated and cut. According to the elevation you give to the hair, you will accomplish a different length, and therefore, a different hairstyle. It is important that you learn how to measure elevations and know how to use them when cutting hair.

When you lift the hair from the scalp, you make an angle. An angle is measured in degrees. To cut hair you will form an angle with the scalp and the hair. The separation between the scalp and the hair will mark the degrees of the angle.

The following figures show the angles that you will use in the cutting technique explained in Chapter II. The small round symbol next to the numbers means degree.

Look at *fig. 1.18.* The separation between these two lines is a ninety-degree angle, (90º.)

Fig. 1.19 shows a forty-five-degree angle (45º) which is one half of the 90º angle.

A 180 degree angle (180º) is a straight line; two 90º angles added together. See *fig. 1.20.*

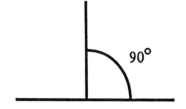

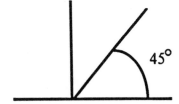

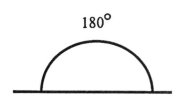

Fig 1.18   *Fig. 1.19*   *Fig. 1.20*

If you are told to elevate the hair at a 90º angle there are two things you need to remember:

1. Think of an imaginary line, or place a ruler touching the head at the base of the hair you are holding. *Fig. 1.21.*

2. Elevate the hair at a 90º angle from this line. If you have difficulty doing this, place your hand flat on the scalp with a strand of hair between your fingers. Lift your hand straight out from this point and you will have a 90º angle.

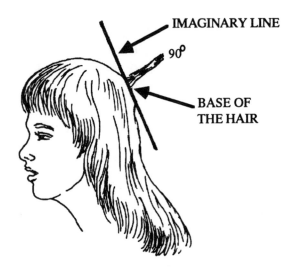

Fig. 1.21

Note that when you elevate the hair at a 90º angle the hair seems to come straight out from the scalp. *Fig. 1.22.*

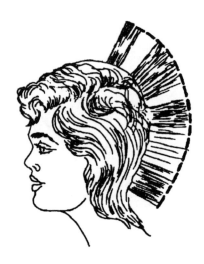

Fig. 1.22

Practice the same method elevating the hair at a 45º angle. See *fig. 1.23.*

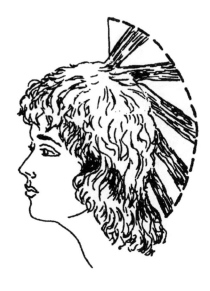

Fig. 1.23

If you are told to elevate the hair at a 180º angle, you will hold it straight up to coincide with the top half of the imaginary line as in *fig. 1.24.*

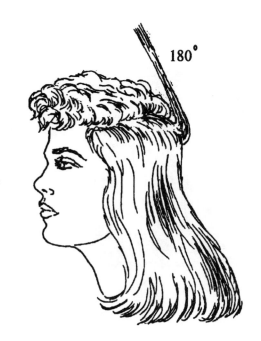

Fig. 1.24

If you look at *fig. 1.25*, you can see a combination of all the angles discussed and how they relate to each other.

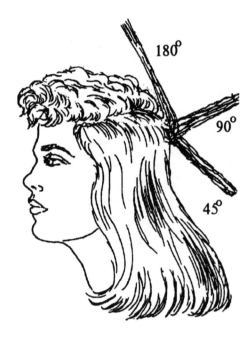

Fig. 1.25

Another term we need to mention is "zero elevation." When you are told to hold the hair at zero elevation, (0º,) keep the hair close to the person's body (occipital bone, neck or back.) Hair that is cut at zero elevation has no layers. This hair is called "one-length." *Fig. 1.26.*

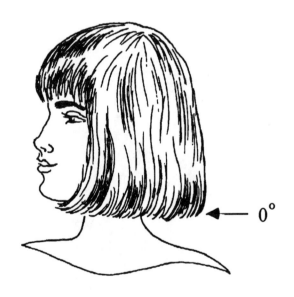

ZERO ELEVATION

Fig. 1.26

30

E. PARTS OF THE HEAD

These terms indicate the parts of the head; they are mentioned in the Sections that follow. Please be familiar with them. *Fig. 1.27.*

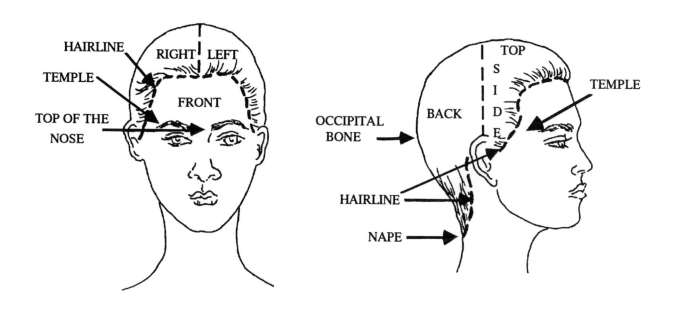

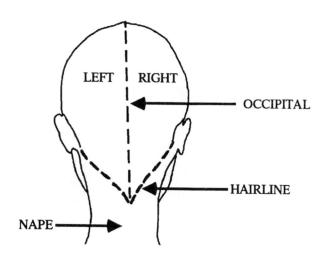

Fig. 1.27

31

F. A WORD ABOUT GUIDES

This section of the book will give you an overview of the guides used in the cutting technique explained in Chapter II. Be familiar with these definitions. As the study progresses you will be able to relate this information to the actual cutting technique. Refer to this section whenever you have questions about the guides.

Guides are points of reference to help you determine the length of each layer being cut. In symmetrical cuts, *see fig 1.28,* guides will also help you determine if the lengths are equally long on either side of the head.

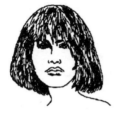
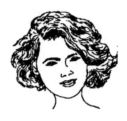

SYMMETRICAL
SIDES HAVE EQUAL LENGTHS

ASSYMETRICAL
SIDES HAVE DIFFERENT LENGTHS

Fig. 1.28

The technique explained in Chapter II employs the following guides:

Outline or perimeter: The perimeter is the edge of the haircut. *Fig. 1.29.* It sets the length and shape that the hair is to have around the face and the back.

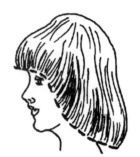
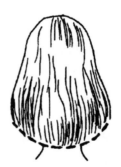
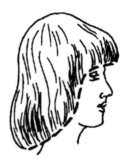
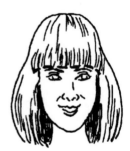

THE BROKEN LINE INDICATES THE PERIMETER

Fig. 1.29

Once the perimeter's length and shape have been defined, it can be elevated at a forty-five-degree or a ninety-degree angle to serve as an initial guide to length of the hair above it. In this way you will give layers to the hair. *Fig. 1.30.*

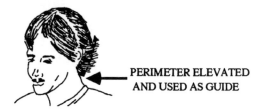

PERIMETER ELEVATED
AND USED AS GUIDE

Fig. 1.30

Hairline: When cutting the outline you will want to leave a distance from the hairline to the perimeter. Never cut above the hairline unless you are giving an exotic haircut. For a very short haircut you can cut at hairline level in the back and the sides. However, in the front you'll have to be careful. If you cut too close to the hairline the cut will look odd, or the hair may stick up. *Fig. 1.31.*

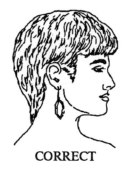
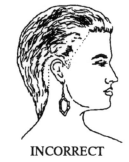

CORRECT   INCORRECT

Fig 1.31

Checkpoints: The purpose of the checkpoint is to indicate the right length to give to the layers before you start cutting sections. It will save you having to retrace your steps and cut more if you left the hair too long, or the possibility of cutting the hair too short, an irreversible mistake.

For example, some types of hair such as straight coarse oriental hair need to have enough length to make the hair heavier--the weight will keep it from sticking up. Other types such as thinning hair need to be cut short enough to produce the volume and bounce it needs or it will lay flat making the scalp visible.

There are two checkpoints: crown-level checkpoint and top-level checkpoint.

Crown-level checkpoint is a one-quarter inch strand of hair located in the center of the crown. Sometimes in the midst of a cowlick or cowlicks. It serves as a guide to determine the length of top, side, and back layers. You will use it in all layered haircuts such as the one-level, bi-level with long-layered back and long-layered styles.

To make this checkpoint, cut the ends of one-quarter inch strand of crown hair and drop it, *see fig. 1.32.* When this hair curls the ends must touch the back of the head. If it is cut too short it will stick up; if too long, it will lay flat. You can easily determine the right length by cutting the ends a bit at a time and dropping the hair to see how it curls. If you still have problems to determine where to cut the crown-level checkpoint, place your comb flat on top of the head; the point where the head separates from the comb will indicate where the checkpoint must be located. *Fig. 1.33.*

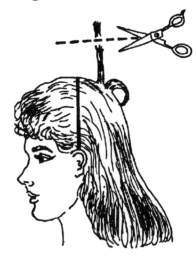
Fig. 1.32

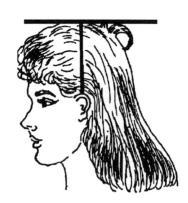
Fig. 1.33

Top-level checkpoint is a one-quarter inch strand of hair located on the top, at joining point of ear-to-ear parting. It will be your guide to determine the length of top and side layers.

This checkpoint is used in haircuts that will be layered on the top only, or on the top and sides with one-length in the back. Haircuts such as bi-level with Bob back, Bob variation, and Bob with one-level top will have the top-level checkpoint. If you give this checkpoint the right length, the hair will curl and bounce touching the crown of the head. *Fig. 1.34.*

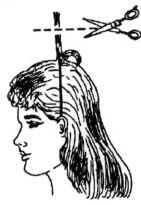
Fig. 1.34

Shoulders: Help to indicate the back lengths. Above the shoulders is a good length for a bob. *Fig. 1.35.*

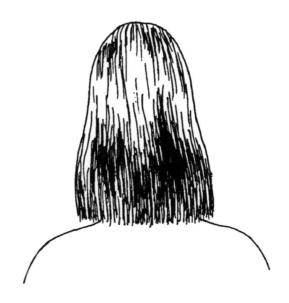

Fig. 1.35

Eyebrows: Help determine the front length. According to the style desired you will cut above the eyebrows, eyebrow level or below the eyebrows. *Fig. 1.36.*

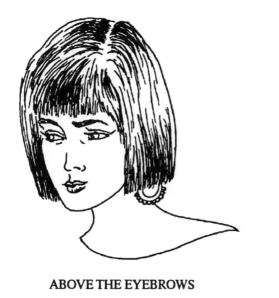 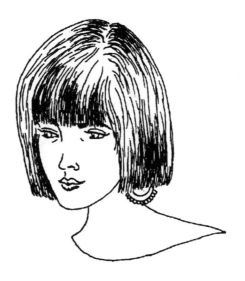

ABOVE THE EYEBROWS   BELOW THE EYEBROWS

Fig. 1.36

35

Mouth, jaw or chin: Serve to indicate top or side lengths. *Fig. 1.37.*

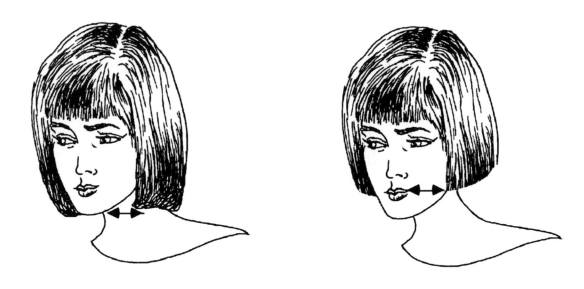

Fig. 1.37

Temples: When the hair is very short in the front and sides, they serve as joining point of front and side outline. To give more length to the hair, cut it below the temples. Also the temples serve as a guide to make the triangle parting on the top. *Fig. 1.38.*

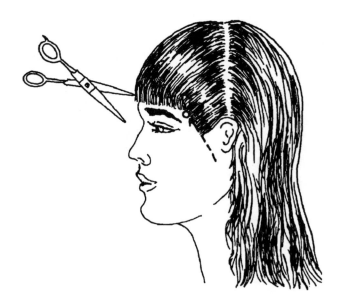

Fig. 1.38

Ears: Serve as a guide to length on both sides of the face. Example: above the ears, mid-ear, and below the ears are common lengths for the side hair. *Fig. 1.39.*

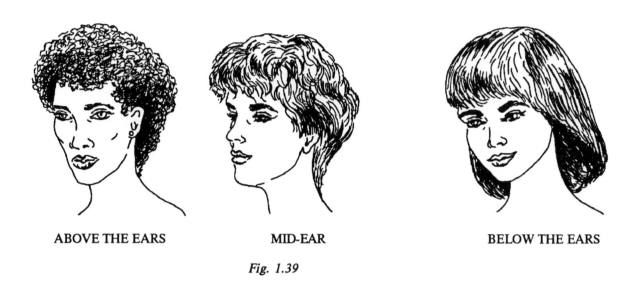

ABOVE THE EARS   MID-EAR   BELOW THE EARS

Fig. 1.39

Nose: Helps you center the top layer and determine the front length. Example: the top, the bridge, and the tip of the nose are common lengths for the front hair. *Fig. 1.40.*

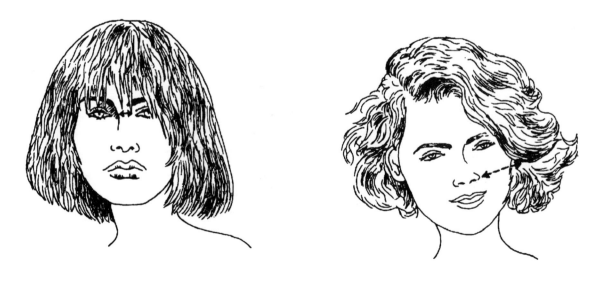

Fig. 1.40

Top layer: Serves as guide to the length of side and back layers. *Fig. 1.41.*

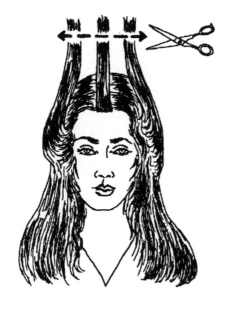

Fig. 1.41

Occipital bone: Serves as a guide to indicate where to stop layering a Wedge haircut. It also serves to indicate the back partings of a Bob haircut. *Fig. 1.42.*

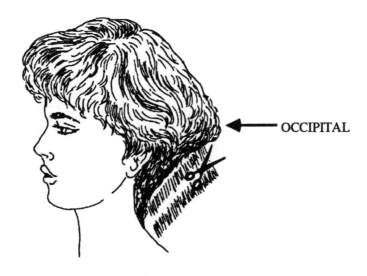

OCCIPITAL

Fig. 1.42

Sections and layers: Sections are divisions within the partings. *Fig. 1.43.* They are approximately one to two inches wide. Some beginners feel that smaller sections are easier to cut, others say that larger sections help them follow the guide better. With smaller sections more precision will be accomplished. When you elevate the section at a chosen degree and cut it, each hair will have a different length. Each length is a layer, *see fig. 1.44.* Sections can be cut in any direction and at any degree according to the desired effect of the final cut. To make clean sections, comb the hair down, part the section, and comb the hair at either side in a horizontal direction. *Fig. 1.44.*

Starting from the second consecutive section, include one-quarter inch of hair from the previous completed section. This quarter inch will not be cut again; it will be a guide to length to your new section. With this procedure you'll be overlapping and blending the sections and you won't miss any hair. *Fig. 1.43.*

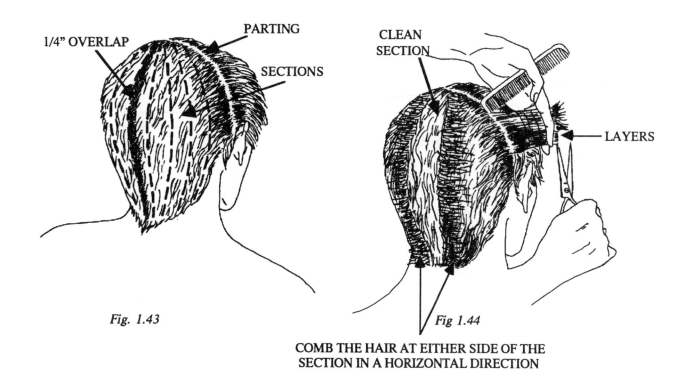

Fig. 1.43

Fig 1.44

COMB THE HAIR AT EITHER SIDE OF THE
SECTION IN A HORIZONTAL DIRECTION

On page thirty we spoke about zero elevation. A sequence of horizontal sections are made to cut the hair at zero elevation; this way it is easier to follow the guide to the length. The technique to cut horizontal sections of hair will be detailed in Chapter II. You can make and use your own points of reference to help yourself accomplish a well balanced haircut. Be aware of your guides and always follow them.

G. LEARN YOUR INCHES

A person's perception of one inch could range from one-quarter of an inch to three inches. To understand as clearly as possible what the person wants, you will show him with your fingers how much hair you are planning to cut, making sure this is what he wants.

Exercise

Place your thumb and index fingers at each end of the different lines on the figure below. Lift your hand trying to keep the separation between the fingers and observe. Now start all over again, this time without looking at the lengths try to duplicate them. Then match the separation of your fingers to the length chosen. Repeat until you can perfectly match the lengths. *Fig. 1.45.*

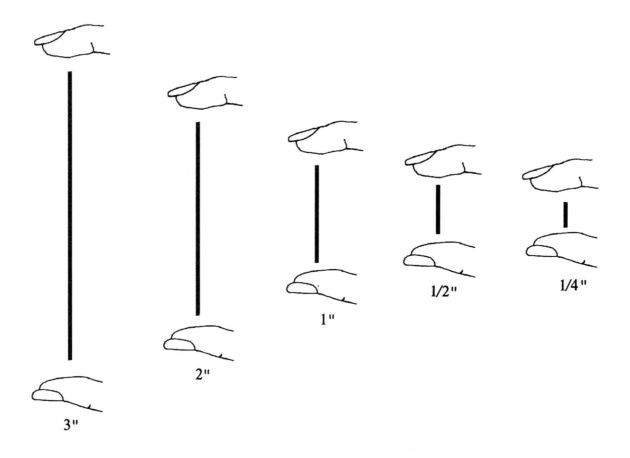

3"   2"   1"   1/2"   1/4"

Fig. 1.45

H. CORRECTIVE HAIRCUTTING

Most people want a haircut that harmonizes with their personality and life-style but it may not suit their type of hair. For example, they may have a picture of a haircut that requires thick hair with body, but their hair is limp; or they may show you a cut for straight hair, but they have super-curly hair. This is when you should explain the limitations that their type of hair imposes. They need to accept what Nature has given them, and find an acceptable style that will enhance their good features.

The first step is to adapt the haircut to the form, texture, and density of the hair. You will have to find out if they are willing to dedicate time to styling the hair to accomplish a desired look, or if they want a wash-and-wear haircut with minimum up-keep. If they are going to change the form of the hair with a permanent wave or a hair straightener, it will be best to give the haircut after the hair has been chemically treated. Also, check the condition of the hair; if the hair is damaged she may want you to cut it shorter to eliminate as much damaged hair as possible.

Note that the form and texture of the hair will determine the appropriate length and haircut, for example:

The best haircuts for straight to wavy hair with thin to medium texture are: one-level, Bob, Bob variations, bi-level with Bob back, and Wedge haircuts.

The best haircuts for wavy, curly, and super-curly hair with medium to thick texture are: one-level, bi-level with long-layered back, and long-layered haircuts.

If the hair has been chemically treated the same haircuts will be acceptable but when cutting it, stretch the hair with less tension to avoid breakage. Also, be gentle when washing it, and select products with mild ingredients.

Once the hair has been washed, observe the following:

1. Natural part of the hair: Wet the hair, comb it straight to the back, and watch it as it naturally parts. When cutting and styling hair with a part on the side, follow the hair's natural movement. Observe that the natural parting connects to the cowlick.

2. Natural direction of the hair: Cowlicks located at the crown give direction to the hair. The direction is more noticeable in short hair. Long hair is directed at the base by its growth pattern, but the longer the hair, the less direction it will show--it has more weight and bends downward. To check the individual pattern of long hair, lift the hair with a comb (do not stretch or pull the hair) and note its direction one half inch from its base. Also examine the cowlick located at the crown and observe its growth pattern.

If the top and side hair tend to go down as it is common in straight hair, cut it short enough to reduce the weight and add volume; if the hair grows toward the back, common in wavy hair, leave it long enough to keep it from sticking up when you comb it back. On pages 155-156, you will find details about how to help give direction to the top hair.

If there is a double cowlick (one next to the other in the crown area, as shown in *fig. 1.46,)* the hair will have more tendency to stick up. Make sure to give the right length to the checkpoint and cut the hair with no tension. If you cut the hair with tension the layers will be uneven due to the different growth patterns in that area. Other cowlicks in hairline areas give direction to the hair of the front, back, or sides. *Fig. 1.47.*

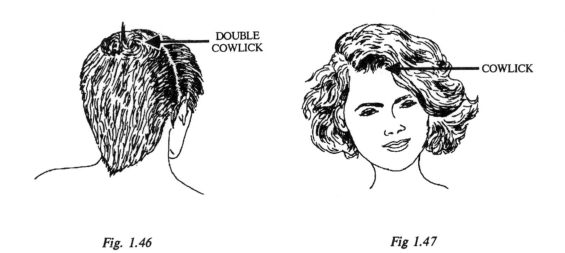

Fig. 1.46   Fig 1.47

The second step is to recommend the appropriate cut to the shape of the face, height, weight and life-style of the person, to obtain the most satisfying haircut. Many people won't care about this factor and only want what they think looks better or feels more comfortable. If that is the case, you will do what the person wants. With experience you will be able to make any length and form of hair work well with any facial shape.

Observe the person, the face, and hairstyle. Visualize the changes that would improve her features. Is the face long or wide? A long face needs some fullness at the sides. Move the hair around, bring it to the sides and observe the effect. Lift the hair in the back. Does a bare neck look better? A wide face needs fullness in the top. Again, move the hair around and observe the different effects accomplished. Make sure to discuss your observations with the individual.

There are seven major facial shapes which are: oval, round, oblong, square, heart, diamond, and triangular.

Oval Face

The oval is considered to be the preferred facial shape. You can make a variety of haircuts on an oval shaped face and they will all look good. Through haircutting you will try to bring each facial shape as close to the oval as possible. However, if the person is overweight with an oval face, there will be corrections to be made. According to your observations you may want to cut the hair medium length and give it volume to make the face appear smaller, or leave it long and layer it to make the face appear longer.

Exercise: Use a pencil first to draw the hair around these faces. Once you've drawn a suitable hair design, go over it with a black marker. Visualize which area of the face needs to be covered or exposed, and where the head should have more or less volume to make the faces look attractive. Follow the suggestions indicated for each facial shape, but don't be afraid to get exotic if you want to. This exercise will help you look at faces with a new perspective. *Fig. 1.48.*

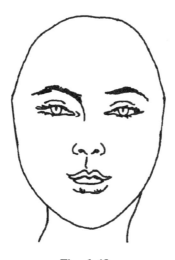

Fig. 1.48

Round Face

The round face needs to look longer and with less fullness in the cheeks. To correct a round shaped face give volume to the top, leave the sides long over the ears, and bring the hair forward towards the cheeks. Since the round face usually has a short forehead, bangs should be short and layered or no bangs at all. Best haircuts: one-level, Bob variation, long-layered. *Fig. 1.49.*

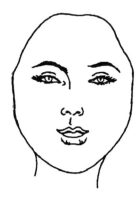

Fig 1.49

Oblong Face

This face is long and narrow, therefore it needs to look wider and shorter. The hair should be short on top with little volume and full on the sides. Bangs or a fringe of bangs to camouflage the forehead should make the face appear shorter. The length of the hair should be short to medium (long hair will make the face look longer). Best haircuts: one-level, Bob variation, bi-levels (sides with volume), and Wedge. *Fig. 1.50.*

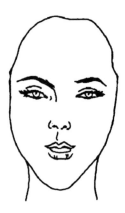

Fig 1.50

Square Face

The goal is to make the face look longer and to smooth the jawbone. The hairstyle requires fullness on top, bangs or a fringe of bangs, and layers to the sides. The length should cover the structure of the jaw. Best haircuts: long-layered, Bob variation, Bob with layered top. *Fig. 1.51.*

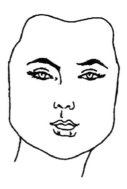

Fig. 1.51

Heart Face

The forehead is wide, the jaw is narrow and round. The hair should be long to smooth the jaw line. Bangs will help hide a wide forehead. Parting the hair on the side will make the head look less wide on top. Best haircuts: Bob, long-layered, bi-levels. *Fig. 1.52.*

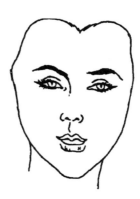

Fig. 1.52

Diamond Face

The forehead and jawbone are narrow, the cheekbones are high, the overall look of the face is long. The forehead should be covered by bangs or a fringe of bangs, and the cheekbones should be smoothed with hair on the sides. Avoid exposing hairline and ears. Best haircuts: long-layered, one-level, Bob variation, Wedge. *Fig. 1.53.*

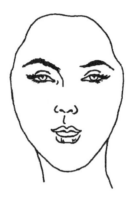

Fig. 1.53

Triangular Face

The forehead is narrow and the jawbone and chin are wide. You need to make the forehead look wider by giving volume to the top. The jawbone can be smoothed with hair around the face. Also, a side parting with the hair combed towards the back, avoiding to expose the entire forehead, and short length helps this facial shape look better. Best haircuts: one-level, Bob variation, bi-levels. *Fig. 1.54.*

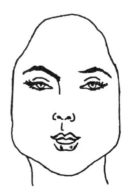

Fig. 1.54

Long hair and flat tops should be avoided if the person is short. Long hair however, suits tall people. Hair that is combed away from the face will accentuate cheekbones and eyes. Towards the face the main focus is on the nose and mouth. These are only general factors to consider. Each person has different characteristics that you must examine and resolve.

Profiles

When analyzing the individual to recommend an appropriate haircut, make sure you also pay attention to her profile. Observe how these have been improved by shaping the hair correctly. The goal is to make the concave and convex look straight. *Fig. 1.55.*

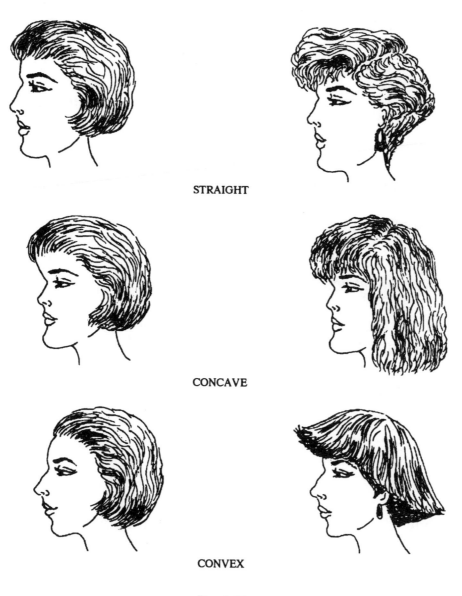

STRAIGHT

CONCAVE

CONVEX

Fig. 1.55

I. BEFORE MAKING THE CUT

Ask the following questions to make sure there is an understanding of what the individual wants and what you can do to his hair. These questions should be asked before every haircut. Promoting this practice will ensure satisfaction at the end of the haircut. Be sure to memorize them.

1. How long ago was your last haircut and did you like it?

This first question will give you a clue as to how long the hair has grown since the last haircut. If the answer is one month, you can assume that the hair has grown approximately one-half inch, therefore, you'll only trim it. However, if the person did not like it because it was left too long or too short, you'll cut either more or less than one-half inch.

2. How short do you want your length in the back?

Ask the person to show you how much she wants cut. If she has long hair she can bring it forward and show you exactly what she wants cut off. Don't start cutting until you know exactly what the person wants.

3. How short would you like the sides? Above the ear, mid-ear, or longer?

Show the length by pointing to your ear and let him show you exactly where he wants his length.

4. How short would you like the top?

Lift the hair at the top with your fingers, look at its length. Does she want the layers short and close to the scalp or does she want fullness?

5. Do you want your hair one-length or layered?

Have her show you where she wants the layers. On the top and sides, on the top only, or all over? Explain what "one-length" means. Make sure you understand how she wants her haircut.

Now that you have clearly established what the subject has in mind in terms of length and style, do not cut it any shorter. In the beginning it is best to be conservative. If you leave the hair longer you can always go back and cut more, but once it is cut too short, only time can correct your error.

Chapter II

TECHNIQUE

Now that you have learned about the tools and the hair, memorized basic terminology, and completed the exercises, you are prepared to learn the technique.

To learn a technique is important to every haircutter. It means that you know where to make your guides and how to follow them--the guides will help you blend the layers and shape the hair in the style desired. You will work in a methodical organized way, gradually moving from a starting to an ending point. This method will increase your efficiency, allowing you to complete a perfect haircut in less time.

In this chapter you will learn how to cut seven different popular haircuts. The primary haircuts are the one-level, the Bob, and the long-layered. By combining these, other styles are obtained. (The Wedge stands on its own.) There are countless variations not included in this book, but with knowledge and practice of this technique, you will be able to cut them.

To be familiar with the looks of each style, see their picture and read their description in the corresponding page for that haircut. The haircuts are: one-level page 65; Bob, page 76; Bob variation, page 93; Bi-level with Bob back, page 101; bi-level with long-layered back, page 113; long-layered, page 126; and Wedge, page 139.

These haircuts are composed of four major steps:

Parting the hair is the first step. All the sample styles are parted in the same fashion except for the back of the head. The back is parted in three different ways depending on whether the hair is to be a one-length, a layered, or a Wedge haircut.

The outline or perimeter is the second step. The outline will be started and ended the same way for all haircuts. According to the style to be cut, you will change the length of the outline where necessary.

Layering is the third step. There are three methods to make layers, 1) for short hair, 2) for long hair, and 3) for the Wedge haircut. One-length haircuts do not require this step.

Checking is the fourth and last step. There are three methods, 1) for short layers, 2) for long layers, and 3) for one-length haircuts.

To remember the steps of each haircut you can try the following methods: 1) answer the questions at the end of each section; if there is something you forgot, look it up, 2) review the technique and jot down the steps of each haircut, 3) read the technique and have a friend ask you to list the steps of each haircut, making sure you don't miss any, 4) record the steps to the haircuts in a tape player and listen to it several times, 5) watch the videotape *"Haircutting Basics"* (refer to the Appendix for information on how to obtain it.) With this videotape you will learn the steps quickly. The goal is to follow the steps automatically from beginning to end of the haircut. Only then, you will be able to concentrate on following the guides and creating the desired look.

Now, read carefully the steps to follow, and get a clear understanding of the haircutting technique before you start the actual cutting. Afterwards you may wish to practice on a friend or a wig.

A. PARTING THE HAIR

Parting the hair refers to the division of the hair into main portions. It is important to distribute the hair to organize your sections and guides as required by the size of the head, bone structure, and intended hair design.

Before the hair is parted it should be washed and untangled. Be sure to maintain the hair wet throughout the haircut.

One-level, bi-level with long-layered back, long-layered, and Wedge haircuts should be parted as explained below. To part a Bob, a bi-level with Bob back, and a Bob variation, see Section D, pages 77-78.

1. Top parting: center, from the crown to the forehead. *Fig. 2.1.*

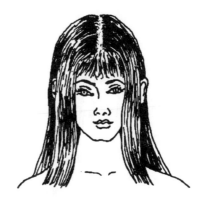

Fig. 2.1

2. Side parting: from ear-to-ear. *Fig. 2.2.*

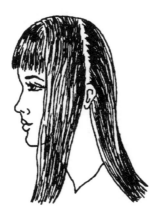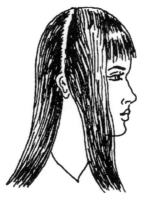

Fig. 2.2

3. Front parting: triangle, from one-third of the top to the temples. *Fig. 2.3.*

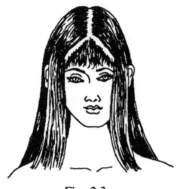

Fig. 2.3

4. Back:

a) Layered cuts: smooth the hair down with no partings. *Fig. 2.4.*

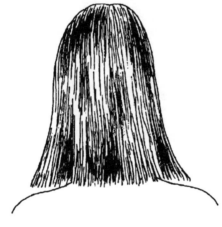

Fig. 2.4

b) Wedge: make V parting from the top of the ears to the occipital bone. *Fig. 2.5.*

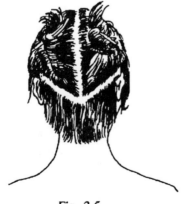

Fig. 2.5

B. THE OUTLINE

The outline is the perimeter that serves as an edge to define the surrounding lengths of the haircut. This edge can have any shape or length desired. The outline is always cut at **zero** elevation.

The outline is composed of four areas: (1) back, (2) front, (3) left side, (4) right side. Eventually you will be cutting it with the hair flat on the skin. Now, to avoid accidental cuts, place the hair between your fingers and stretch it at zero elevation. Cut with the scissors close to the fingers on the palm side of your hand.

a) To Outline the Back: one-level, bi-level with long-layered back, long-layered, and Wedge.

Note: To outline a Bob and Bob variation see page 76. To outline a bi-level with Bob back see page 101.

<u>From the center of the back to the left side</u>

1. After discussing with the subject the desired length and hairstyle, part the hair accordingly. See illustrations in Section A, pages 51-52.

2. Tilt the subject's head forward to avoid tapering the outline and to have a comfortable position for cutting. If you are outlining a Wedge make sure the hair is short. If the hair is below the nape the ends will flip up.

3. Comb the hair of the back free of tangles.

4. Hold a one-inch wide section of hair from the center of the back. Slide your fingers to the point where you want to cut. Keep the fingers near the blades to cut in a straight line. *Fig. 2.6.*

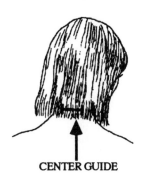

CENTER GUIDE

Fig. 2.6

5. Cut toward the left side in small snips with the tips of the scissors. Do not cut beyond the second joint of the index finger. Only the hair stretched between the first two joints pulls the hair with even tension.

6. Snip five times, stop, comb, and make a new section including one-quarter inch of the section previously cut as a guide to the length. Do not cut the guide, only continue extending the line from the center.

7. Cut slowly and stand back at times to observe how is your outline coming along.

8. Once you cut the left side of the back in a straight line, comb the hair again, go back to the starting point, and check if your line is straight and clean; if it is not, cut where needed only. Do not cut the hair shorter than you had planned. If your line is not perfectly straight leave it as it is or you may cut it too short. With practice your line will be perfect. *Fig. 2.7.*

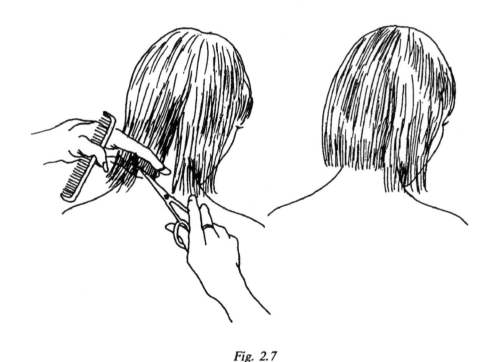

Fig. 2.7

Now, the left side of the back outline is completed. Breath deeply and get ready to start cutting the right side of the back. To cut it easily and accurately, break the line in two sections. This way you'll have the guide visible at all times as explained in the proceeding steps.

From the center of the back to the right side

1. Tilt the subject's head forward.

2. Start in the middle of the right section and cut towards the center. *Fig. 2.8*

3. Cut section two and join it with section one. *Fig. 2.9.*

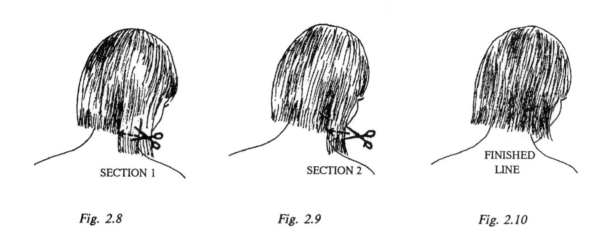

| SECTION 1 | SECTION 2 | FINISHED LINE |

Fig. 2.8   *Fig. 2.9*   *Fig. 2.10*

b) To Outline the Front

The front outline may have any shape you want. It can be cut straight, longer in the middle or shorter in the middle. In the sample haircut the front outline will be cut shorter in the middle. *Fig. 2.11.*

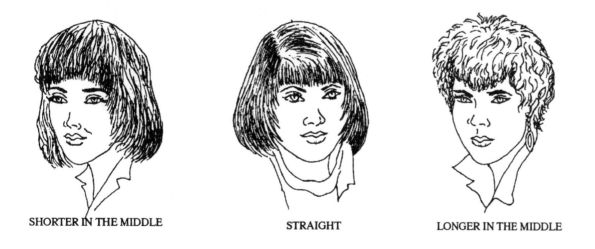

SHORTER IN THE MIDDLE   STRAIGHT   LONGER IN THE MIDDLE

Fig. 2.11

Usually eyebrow level or longer is a good length for the front outline. Remember that cowlicks and widow's peaks are common in the front hairline, so keep an eye for them.

From the center of the front to the right temple

1. Lift the subject's head straight.

2. Stand in front of the subject.

3. Re-adjust the front parting.

4. Cut a center guide on top of the nose. *Fig. 2.12.*

5. Cut from the center guide to the right temple in a downward direction. *Fig. 2.13.* To give extra length to the front hair, cut below the temple.

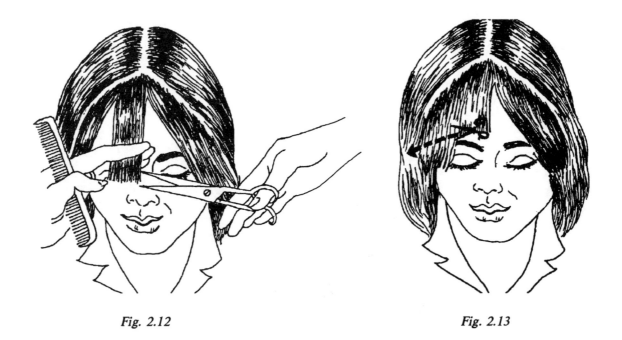

Fig. 2.12   *Fig. 2.13*

Now the right side is completed. Breath deeply and get ready to cut the left side.

<u>From the center of the front to the left temple</u>

The left side of the front outline will be parted in two sections. This way you'll always have your guide visible.

1. Cut the first section and join it with the center guide. *Fig. 2.14.*

2. Cut the second section in an upward direction from the left temple to section one and join them. Make sure that you place your fingers in the same angle you had them on the right side. *Fig. 2.15.*

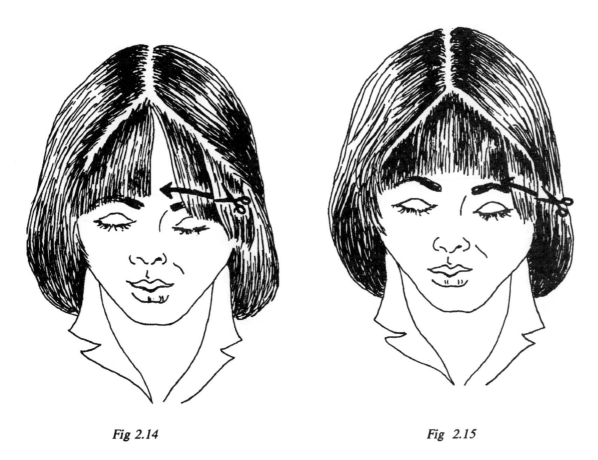

Fig 2.14   Fig 2.15

3. Once the left side is finished stand back and observe. Make the necessary adjustments.

Do you have an even curvature? Is the hair too short, too long? If the hair is too long make a new guide in the center and start again. Adjustments should be made cutting one-quarter inch at a time. Remember that once the hair dries it will be shorter.

To outline the sides of a long-layered haircut turn to page 60.

c) To Outline the Sides: short hair (one-level, bi-level, Wedge).

<u>Left Side</u>

1. Stand next to the subject's left side.

2. Re-establish ear-to-ear parting.

3. Tilt the subject's head to the right side.

4. Comb the hair down over the ear. *Fig. 2.16.*

5. Cut the side length in a straight line from the ear to the cheek. Do not cut above the hairline. *Fig. 2.16.*

6. Comb all the hair of the left side towards the front. *Fig. 2.17.*

7. Cut in an upward direction toward the temple and meet the frontal outline. Make sure to drop the outline. *Fig. 2.17.*

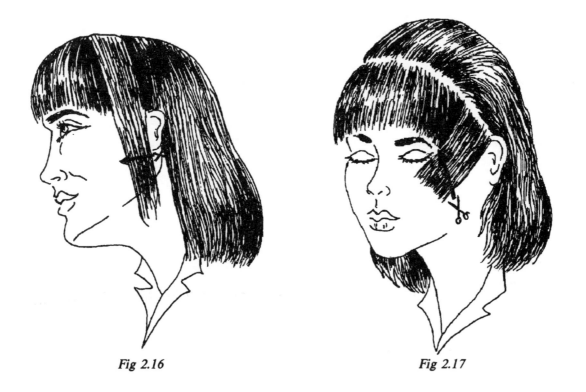

Fig 2.16   *Fig 2.17*

Now the left side is completed. Get ready to cut the right side.

Right Side

Proceed to outline the right side using the same method.

1. Stand next to the subject's right side.

2. Re-adjust ear-to-ear parting.

3. Tilt the subject's head to the left side.

4. Comb the hair over the ear. *Fig. 2.18.*

5. Cut the same length of the left side. You may use the bones of the ears as points of reference to make sure that both sides have the same length. *Fig. 2.18.*

6. Comb the hair of the right side toward the front. *Fig. 2.19.*

7. Cut in a downward direction from the right temple to the earlobe. *Fig. 2.19.*

8. Breath deeply; stand back and observe.

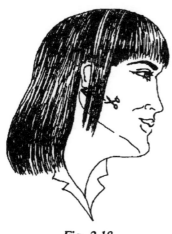

Fig. 2.18

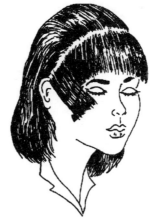

Fig 2.19

Now both sides are completed. To continue and finish the haircuts listed below return to their corresponding Section and page.

One-level: Section C, page 68. Bi-level with long-layered back: Section G, page 117. Wedge: Section I, page 143.

d) To Outline the Sides: long hair (long-layered, Bob variation).

1. If the hair of the sides is below the shoulders and the style is straight, turn the head to the left and align chin over shoulder. Cut the side using the back length as a guide. Cut from the back to the left side. *Fig. 2.20.*

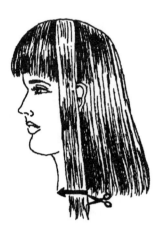

Fig 2.20

To cut the right side, first divide it in two sections; this way you'll have the guide visible at all times.

1. Cut section one to join with the back. *Fig. 2.21.*

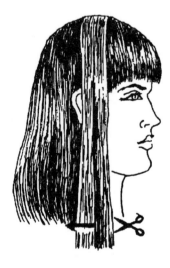

Fig. 2.21

2. Cut section two from the front to section one. *Fig. 2.22.*

3. To check that both sides have equal lengths tilt the head forward and measure with the comb, or meet the ends of the sides in the front. See illustrations on page 63.

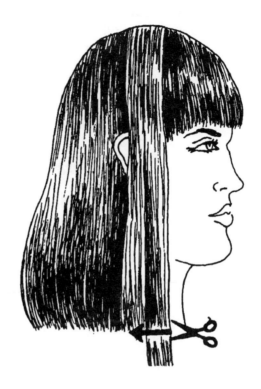

Fig. 2.22

e) To Angle the Sides of Long Hair (long-layered, Bob variation).

If the hair of the sides is long and to be layered, such as in a Bob variation or a long-layered haircut, they may be angled to give graduation to the outline; the result will be a feathery effect on the sides and more movement of the side hair towards the back.

Cut the sides as explained in page 60, Section (d) and proceed as follows:

Place your hand in the angle that you want to cut. Use the bones or features of the face as a guide to the length. If the hair is very long you may want to use other parts of the body as a reference to the length.

61

Left Side

1. Stand facing the subject's left side.

2. Elevate the hair sliding the fingers towards the front. Let outline drop.

3. Cut on the palm side of your hand. *Fig. 2.23.*

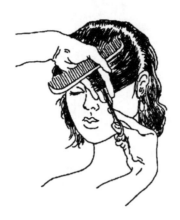

Fig 2.23

Right side

1. Stand behind the subject.

2. Lift the hair towards the front sliding your fingers in a vertical position and cut on the back side of your hand. *Fig. 2.24.*

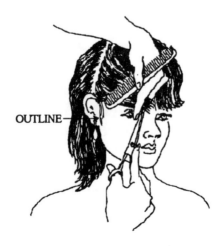

OUTLINE

Fig. 2.24

Now the sides have been angled. Check the lengths as follows:

Tilt the head forward and let the hair of the sides hang. With the comb parallel to the floor measure the sides and make sure they are the same length. *Fig. 2.25.*

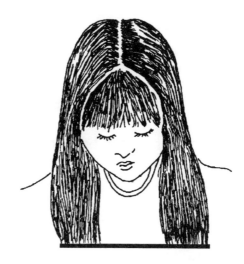

Fig 2.25

Another way to measure the sides is by meeting the side lengths in the front. *Fig. 2.26.*

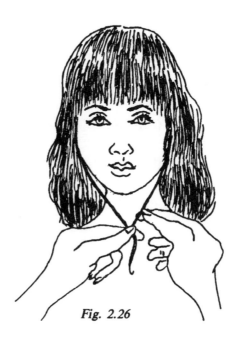

Fig. 2.26

Now the outline is finished. To complete a Bob variation return to Section E, page 96. To complete a long-layered haircut return to Section H, page 130.

REVIEW QUESTIONS

To make sure that you thoroughly understand the steps necessary to cut the outline, answer the following questions. The answers can be found in the page numbers noted at the side.

1. How do the eyebrows and temples help you cut the front outline? pp. 35-36

2. What are some of the different lengths of the side outline? p. 37

3. What would determine the partings to be made before outlining the hair? p. 51

4. What is an outline? p. 53

5. At what degree would you cut the outline? p. 53

6. Where would you start the outline? p. 53

7. What are the three other areas that compose an outline and in what order are they cut? p. 53

8. Why should the head be tilted forward or to the side when the hair is being outlined? p. 53

9. List the sections of the back outline. p. 53

10. List the guides that help you cut the back outline. pp. 53, 55

11. List the sections of the front outline. pp. 56-57

12. List the sections of the left side short outline. p. 58

13. What styles have a short outline on the sides? p. 58

14. List the sections of the right side of a short outline. p. 59

15. How would you outline the sides of long hair? pp. 60-61

16. How would you angle the sides of long hair? pp. 60-62

17. What styles with long hair have angled sides? p. 61

C. ONE-LEVEL

The one-level haircut is an easy-care style, a favorite of many women of all ages and men's classic haircut.

This style can be cut super short or longer. The layers can be shaped to provide volume to the top and length to the back, while the sides can be tapered close to the head. Another variation is with the top long and the sides and the back very short; also, you can keep it short all over framing the face. Just be aware that with the same basic technique, you can accomplish many different looks by adjusting the length of the layers in different areas of the head. *Fig. 2.27.*

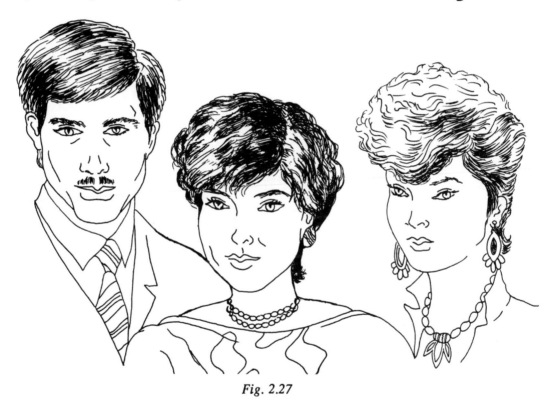

Fig. 2.27

PARTING THE HAIR

See illustrations on Section A, page 51.

Top parting: center, from the crown to the forehead.

Side parting: from ear-to-ear.

Front parting: triangle, from one-third of the top to the temples.

Back: smooth it down with no parting.

GUIDES

The following guides will be used to cut a one-level haircut.

Hairline
Top of the nose
Eyebrows   } OUTLINE
Ears
Perimeter

Crown-level checkpoint
Nose   } LAYERS
Top section
Sections and layers

ANGLES

This style will be cut at a ninety-degree angle. *Fig. 2.28.*

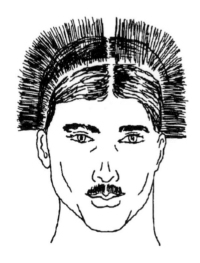 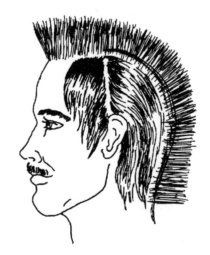

Fig 2.28

LAYERED SECTIONS

Adjust the number of sections according to the size of the head.

Section one corresponds to the top. *Fig. 2.29.*

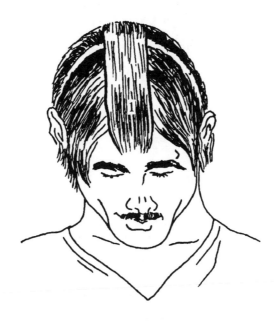

Fig. 2.29

Section two, left side. *Fig. 2.30.*

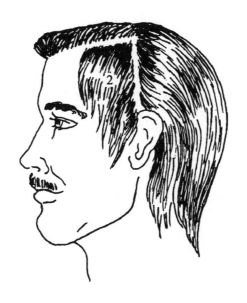

Fig. 2.30

Sections three, four, five, six, and seven, to the back. *Fig. 2.31.*

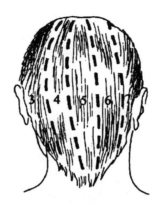

Fig. 2.31

Section eight, right side. *Fig. 2.32.*

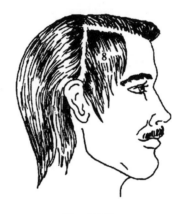

Fig. 2.32

OUTLINE

1. Outline the back, front, and sides. See page 53 for details.

Once the outline is completed, return to this page and proceed to cut the layers as follows:

CUTTING THE LAYERS

Section One: top

1. Stand next to the subject's left side.

2. Cut crown-level checkpoint. See page 34 for details to cut this guide.

3. Comb the top hair forward. *Fig. 2.33.*

4. Make a two-inch wide section from crown-level checkpoint to the front. *Fig. 2.33.*

5. Elevate one-third of the section at a time at a ninety-degree angle. Use the nose as a guide to center section one. *Fig. 2.34.*

6. Cut from crown-level checkpoint to the front perimeter in a straight line. Let the front perimeter drop. *Fig. 2.34.*

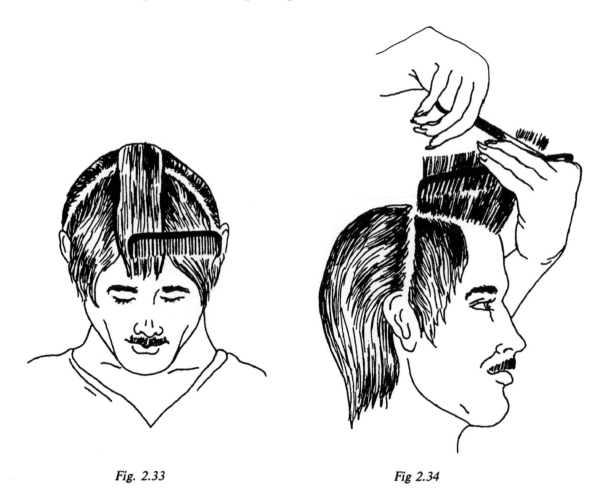

Fig. 2.33   Fig 2.34

Now the top has been completed. Breath deeply and get ready to layer the sides.

Section Two: left side

1. Remain next to the subject's left side. Make a center parting in the the top and re-adjust ear-to-ear parting.

2. Make a straight and vertical side section from the ear to the top.

3. Elevate the perimeter at a ninety-degree angle and use it as the first guide to the length of the layers. Cut this section in vertical direction from the perimeter to the top. *Fig. 2.35.*

4. Snip five times, drop the hair, comb it, take more hair, elevate it and cut again. Always use a one-quarter inch of the layers previously cut as a guide to the length of the next section.

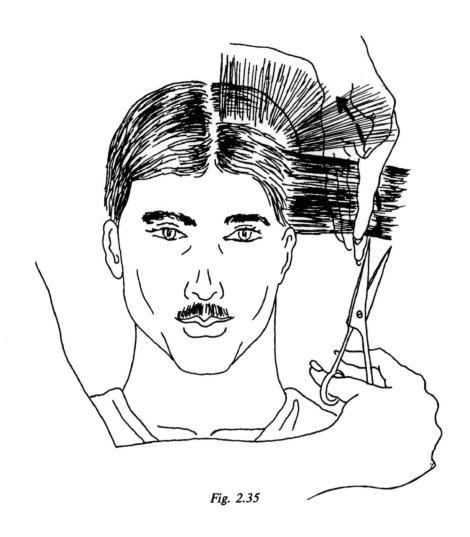

Fig. 2.35

Section Three Through Seven: back

You will need to make more or less sections according to the size of the head. A child's head is smaller than an adult's and since children grow very impatient in a short period of time you need to finish the haircut as fast as you can, therefore, three sections may be enough to cut the layers of the back. A large head however, may need more than five sections. Make adjustments as necessary.

1. Stand next to the subject's left side and move around the back as you approach the left side.

2. Make clean vertical sections, one-and-a-half to two inches wide. Include one-quarter inch from previous sections as a guide to the length.

3. Starting at the hairline elevate the hair at a ninety-degree angle and cut upwards to join the side with the top. *Fig. 2.36.*

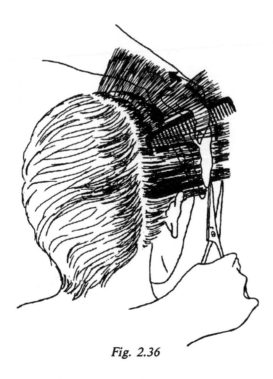

Fig. 2.36

Make sure that your guide is visible at all times with each new section you hold. If you lose your guide stop, define your section and then continue, or bend the ends of the hair as you hold it to see the length of your guide.

4. Repeat the steps adding sections until you get to section eight on the right side.

Section Eight: right side

1. Re-adjust ear-to-ear parting.

2. Stand behind the subject's right shoulder. In this position you should be able to see your guide.

3. Make a section from the ear to the front. Include one-quarter inch of section eight as a guide to the length.

4. Cut from the perimeter to the top. When you elevate section eight do not stretch the hair towards the back. Make sure you are holding the hair at a ninety-degree angle, otherwise this section will be longer than section two on the left side of the head. *Fig. 2.37.*

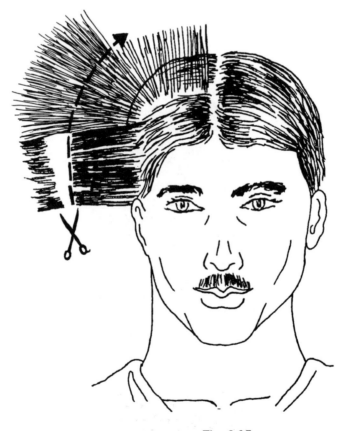

Fig. 2.37

5. Breath deeply; stand back, observe, and get ready to check the haircut.

CHECKING

Once you have cut the last section, the next step is to check the haircut. If the sections are uneven, even them out. Do not make unnecessary cuts and do not make new guides.

Ask yourself if you have made any of the following mistakes; they could be the reasons to uneven lengths of hair in your sections: Did you apply too much tension to some sections? Did you stretch the hair with tension in the cowlick areas? Did you follow the guide at all times? Were some of the sections too large and others too small? Did you make clean partings?

Stand behind the subject and start checking the hair in the following way:

1. Crown: Take a horizontal section at the crown, elevate it at a ninety-degree angle. Ideally this section should be perfectly straight. If it is longer on one side, it indicates that one side of the head has longer hair. In this case start the haircut from the beginning. Otherwise even out the hair and go on to the next step. *Fig. 2.38.*

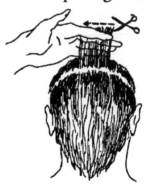

Fig. 2.38

2. Top: Make a section on top and stand behind the subject. Check the hair at a ninety-degree angle in three horizontal sections from the crown to the front. *Fig. 2.39.*

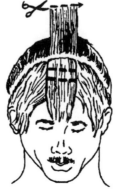

Fig. 2.39

73

3. Sides: Check the sides horizontally starting at the top and working your way down to the hairline. Hold the hair at a ninety-degree angle and cut if necessary to even out the hair. *Fig. 2.40.*

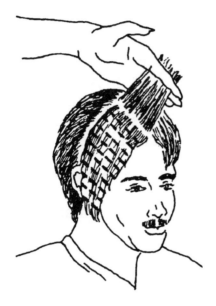

Fig. 2.40

4. Back: Elevate the hair of the crown at a ninety-degree angle. Continue checking the center of the back in horizontal sections until you reach the perimeter. Do the left and the right side of the back from the top to the perimeter. *Fig. 2.41.* If there is hair flipping up behind the ears cut it below the hairline. *Fig. 2.42.*

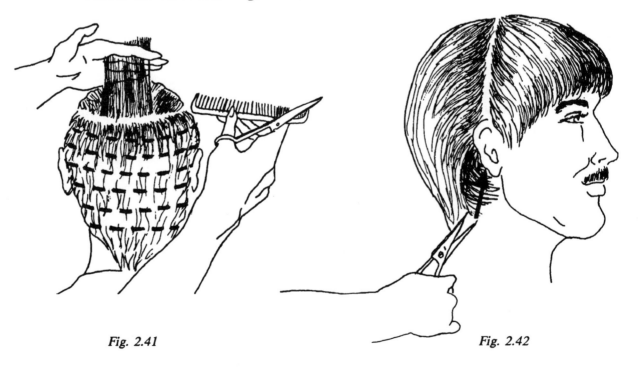

Fig. 2.41   *Fig. 2.42*

REVIEW QUESTIONS

To ensure that you have learned the steps of the one-level haircut, answer the following questions. The page numbers next to the questions indicate where the answers can be found.

1. How can the perimeter be a guide? p. 33

2. Explain what each of the following guides indicate: pp. 32-39
   a) hairline
   b) crown-level checkpoint
   c) nose
   d) top section
   e) sections and layers

3. Why can the crown present problems? p. 42

4. What are the five questions to ask before starting the haircut? p. 48

5. How would you part the hair to cut a one-level style? p. 65

6. At what degree would you elevate the hair to cut a one-level? p. 66

7. List the sections of the one-level haircut. pp. 67-68

8. What would you cut first, the outline or the layers? pg 68

9. Where would you start layering the hair and where would you end the haircut? pp. 69-74

10. In what direction (vertical or horizontal), would you cut side and back layers? p. 70

11. Explain briefly how would you check the top, back, and sides of this haircut. pp. 73-74

12. In what direction would you hold the hair to check it, vertically or horizontally? pp. 73-74

D. BOB

The Bob haircut is a one-length hairstyle excellent for straight hair that needs bounce. Most popular manageable lengths range from jawbone to just above the shoulders. These lengths allow the Bob freedom of movement for a bouncy look and its line will not be disturbed by the hair touching the shoulders. *Fig. 2.43.*

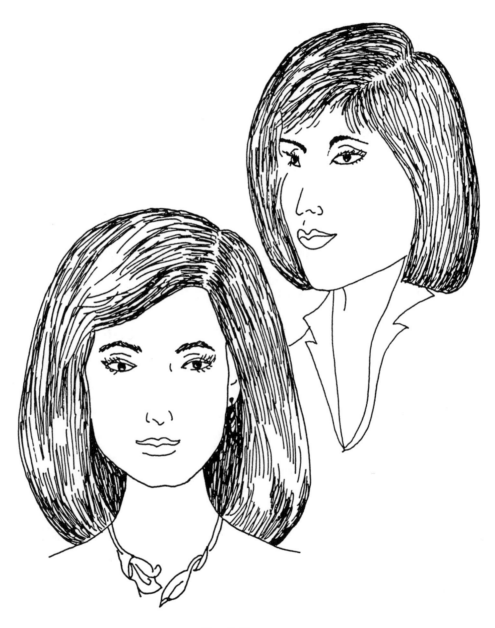

Fig. 2.43

PARTING THE HAIR

Top parting: center, from the crown to the forehead. *Fig. 2.44.*

Some people wear this style with a side parting. If the person is going to wear it parted on the side all the time, you must cut it parted on that side; this way the hair of the top will have the length of the side perimeter. *Fig. 2.45.*

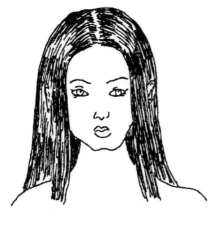

Fig 2.44

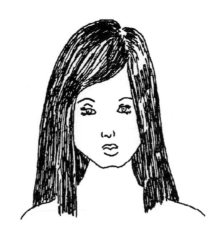

Fig 2.45

Side parting: from ear-to-ear. *Fig. 2.46.*

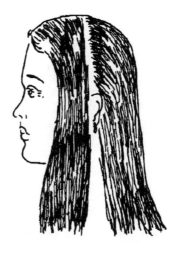

Fig. 2.46

If the hair is very thick, divide the hair in half-horizontals in the following way:

Make a horizontal parting at eye level from ear-to-ear parting to the front. Pin the upper section out of the way and smooth the rest of the hair down. *Fig. 2.47.*

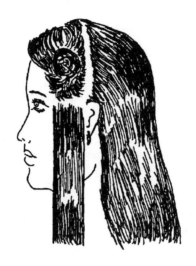

Fig. 2.47

Front parting: for bangs, make triangle parting from one-third of the top to the temples. *Fig. 2.48.*

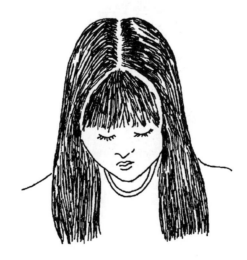

Fig. 2.48

Back parting: triangle, from the occipital bone to below the ears. Pin the upper section out of the way and smooth the rest of the hair down. *Fig. 2.49.*

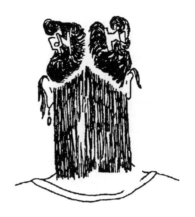

Fig. 2.49

GUIDES

Shoulders
Top of the nose
Back perimeter
Eyebrows
Temples
Sections

ANGLES

The Bob is cut at zero elevation. *Fig. 2.50.*

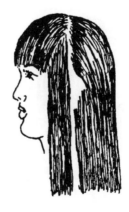

Fig. 2.50

SECTIONS

Sections one, two, and three correspond to the first layer of the back. *Fig. 2.51.*

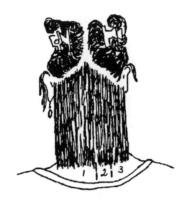

Fig. 2.51

Sections four, five, and six to the second layer of the back. *Fig. 2.52.*

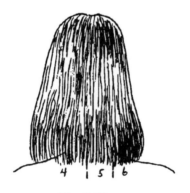

Fig. 2.52

Section seven, left side. *Fig. 2.53.*

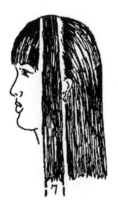

Fig. 2.53

Section eight and nine, right side. *Fig. 2.54.*

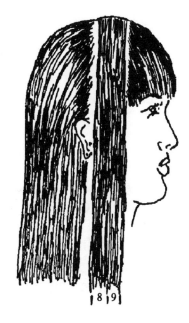

Fig. 2.54

Sections ten, eleven, and twelve, bangs. *Fig. 2.55.*

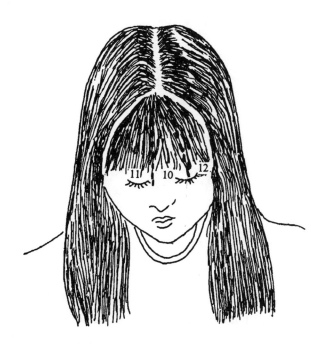

Fig. 2.55

CUTTING THE SECTIONS

BACK

First Layer of the Back
Section One: left side

1. Part the hair.

2. Stand behind the subject.

3. Tilt the subject's head forward and ask her to keep it that way while you cut the back. This way you'll avoid taper in the perimeter.

4. Place a one-inch wide section from the center of the back between the middle and index fingers of your left hand. Slide your fingers to the point where you want to cut. Keep the scissors close to the fingers to keep the line straight.

5. Cut toward the left side in small snips with the tips of the scissors. *Fig. 2.56.* Do not cut beyond the second joint of the index finger, this way you will avoid accidental cuts to your hand and the perimeter will be straight.

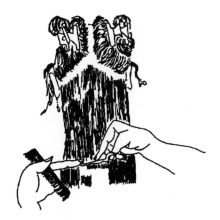

Fig. 2.56

6. Snip five times, stop, comb, take a new section with one-quarter inch of the hair previously cut as a guide to the length. Do not cut the guide, if you do, you'll change the length of the hair; just continue extending the line from the center. Cut slowly and stand back at times to observe.

7. Once you have cut the left side in a straight line, comb the hair again, go back to the starting point, and check if your line is straight and clean. If it is not, cut where needed only.

Do not cut the hair shorter than planned. If your line is not perfectly straight leave it as it is or you may cut it too short. With practice, your lines will be perfect.

Now the left side of the back outline is completed. Breath deeply and get ready to cut the right side of the back outline as explained below:

Sections Two and Three: right side

To cut the perimeter with accuracy divide it in two sections. This way you will have the guide visible at all times.

1. Tilt the subject's head forward.

2. Start in the middle of the right side.

3. Cut section two towards the center guide. *Fig. 2.57.*

4. Move to section three and join it with section two. *Fig. 2.58.*

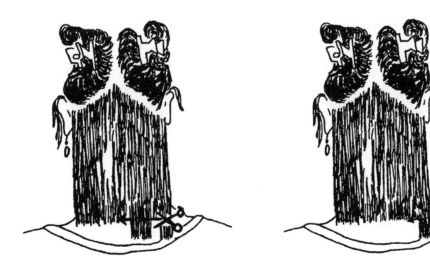

Fig. 2.57   *Fig. 2.58*

Now the back is completed. Get a mirror and show the back length to the person. Make sure this is the length desired. If it's too long make a new guide and cut more, otherwise check the back as follows:

5. Gather the hair in your comb and slide it down from the parting to the perimeter. Place the comb parallel to the floor and check the line. If there are a few wisps of hair hanging, cut them. If the crooked areas are less than one-quarter inch too long, leave the length alone. If there are differences in length of one-half inch or more start from the beginning with a new guide. *Fig. 2.59.*

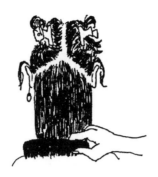

Fig. 2.59

Second Layer of the Back
Section Four: left side

1. Once the first layer of the back is completed bring the rest of the hair down and comb it free of tangles.

2. Tilt the subject's head forward.

3. Cut from the center to the left as you did in the previous layer. This time, roll your fingers down to make this layer slightly longer--the hair will naturally fold under. Follow the length of the first layer as your guide but make sure you are not cutting it. *Fig. 2.60.*

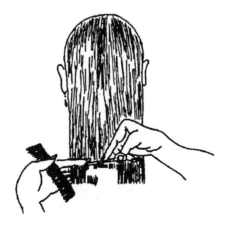

Fig. 2.60

Sections Five and Six: right side

1. Divide the right side in two sections. Use the same procedure of the first layer, but this time, roll the fingers down as indicated in section four.

2. Cut section five and join it to section four. *Fig. 2.61.*

3. Cut from section six to section five and join those two sections. *Fig. 2.62.*

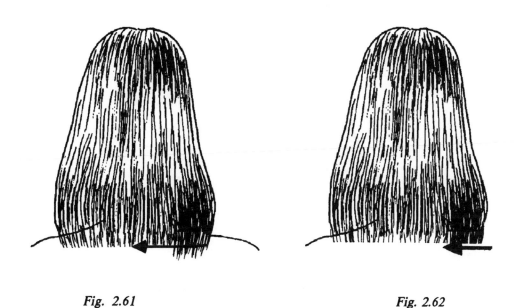

Fig. 2.61   Fig. 2.62

   Now the back has been completed. If you are cutting a bi-level with Bob back, you can now return to Section F, page 108 to complete the haircut. If you are cutting a Bob proceed to the next page to cut the sides.

SIDES
Section Seven: left side

If the sides had thick abundant hair and were parted in half-horizontals, cut the first layer straight and the second layer rolling the fingers down. Otherwise do not roll the fingers to cut the sides. If you are cutting a Bob variation do not roll the fingers down.

1. Move to the subject's left side.

2. Roll the fingers down while you hold the hair and continue cutting the outline towards the left side. *Fig. 2.63.*

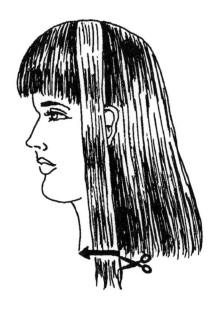

Fig. 2.63

Sections Eight and Nine: right side

1. Stand next to the subject's right side.

An easy accurate method to cut the right side is by breaking the line in two sections to have your guide visible.

2. Cut section eight and join it to the back. *Fig. 2.64.*

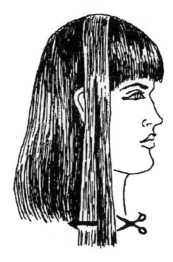

Fig. 2.64

3. Cut section nine from the front to section eight. Stretch the hair at zero elevation while you cut. *Fig. 2.65.*

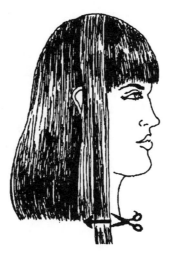

Fig. 2.65

Now the sides are completed. Breath deeply and get ready to cut the front.

FRONT
Section Ten: right side

The front outline may have any shape you want. It can be made straight or angled (longer in the middle or shorter in the middle). In the sample haircut I'll explain how to cut the front outline shorter in the middle.

Usually eyebrow level or longer is a good length for the front outline.

1. Lift the subject's head straight and face the subject.

2. Re-adjust the triangle parting on the front.

3. Hold a one-inch strand of hair in the middle of the forehead.

4. Cut it at zero elevation. This middle strand will be a guide to the length of the front outline. *Fig. 2.66.*

5. Cut section ten from the middle of the front to the right temple in a downward direction. *Fig. 2.67.*

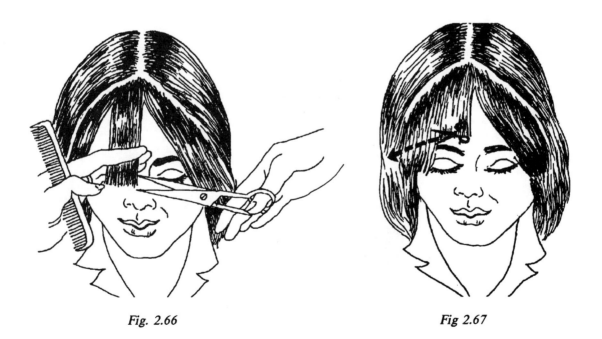

Fig. 2.66   Fig 2.67

Now the right side is completed. Check that the line is straight and get ready to cut the left side.

Sections Eleven and Twelve: left side

The left side of the front outline will be parted in two sections. This way you'll always have your guide visible.

1. Cut section eleven at zero elevation and join it with the center guide. *Fig. 2.68.*

2. Cut section twelve in an upward direction, from the left temple to section eleven and join both sections. *Fig. 2.69.*

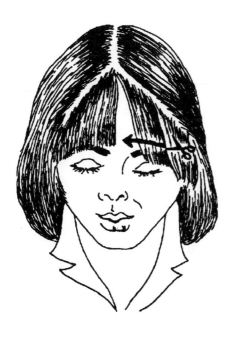

Fig. 2.68

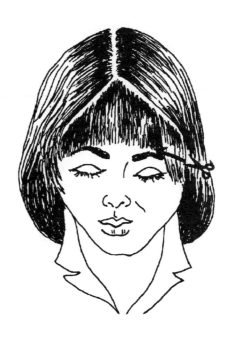

Fig. 2.69

3. Breath deeply; stand back, and observe.

Note: To angle the sides of a Bob variation turn to Section B, page 62.

CHECKING

Once you have cut the last section, the next step is to check the haircut. If there is uneven hair in the sections, cut them even. Do not make unnecessary cuts and do not make new guides.

Ask yourself if you have made any of the following mistakes; they could be the reasons to uneven lengths of hair in your sections: Did you apply too much tension to some sections of hair? Did you follow the guide at all times? Did you maintain the scissors straight with your fingers? Did you tilt the head forward while cutting the back? Did you cut the hair at zero elevation at all times? Now, stand behind the subject and check the haircut in the following way.

1. Back: Gather the hair of the back in your comb and slide it down from the occipital bone to the perimeter. Place the comb parallel to the floor and check the line. If the perimeter is uneven, cut where the lengths are longer. If the length is one-half inch longer on one side, part the hair and start from the beginning. *Fig. 2.70.*

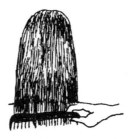

Fig. 2.70

2. Sides: Tilt the subject's head forward and allow the sides to hang. Use your comb to measure or meet the ends in the front to make sure the sides have the same length. *Fig. 2.71.*

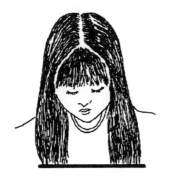 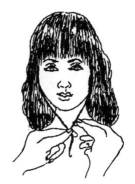

Fig 2.71

Note: To layer the bangs turn to Chapter III, page 153.

How to Cut a One Level Top on a Bob Haircut

1. Part the hair from ear-to-ear.

2. Cut top-level checkpoint. See page 34 for details.

3. Make a triangle section from top-level checkpoint to the temples. *Fig. 2.72*

4. Elevate the section at a ninety-degree angle in a vertical direction. *Fig. 2.73*

5. Cut from the checkpoint to the front. Make sure the perimeter drops uncut. *Fig. 2.73.*

6. Stand behind the subject.

7. Check the hair in three horizontal sections from the checkpoint to the front. *Fig. 2.74.*

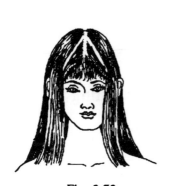

Fig. 2.72

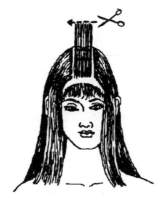

Fig. 2.74

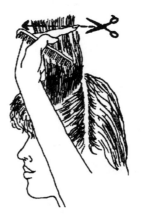

Fig. 2.73

REVIEW QUESTIONS

To ensure that you have learned the steps of the Bob haircut, answer the following questions. The page numbers next to the questions indicate where the answers can be found.

1. Explain how the following guides help you cut a Bob. pp. 32-39
   a) shoulders
   b) temples
   c) sections
   d) eyebrows
   e) back perimeter
   f) top of the nose

2. How would you part the hair to cut a bob? pp. 77-78

3. How would you cut the hair if the person always parts her hair on the side? p. 77

4. What are half-horizontals? p. 78

5. At what degree would you cut a Bob? p. 79

6. Why is it important not to cut into the guides? p. 82

7. Why is it important to tilt the head forward while cutting the back? p. 82

8. Where would you start cutting the sections? p. 82

9. Which is an accurate way to cut the right side of the back? p. 83

10. How would you place your fingers to cut the second layer? p. 84

11. Where would you start cutting the front and in how many sections? pp. 88-89

12. Where would you end the haircut? p. 90

13. How would you part the hair to cut a one-level top? p. 91

14. What guides would you use to cut a one-level top? p. 91

15. At what degree would you cut a one-level top? p. 91

16. In what direction would you check a one-level top? p. 91

E. BOB VARIATION--Bob with one-level top and long-layered sides

    This haircut combines three styles. The back is one-length, the sides are long and layered, the top is short and layered. The layers of the top and sides will bring bounce and volume to wavy hair or a feathered look to straight hair. Through styling, this haircut can be changed into a number of different looks to match a variety of daytime or evening activities. *Fig. 2.75.*

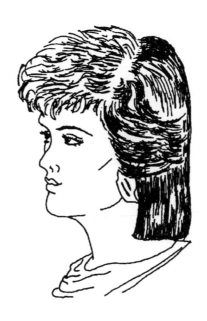

Fig. 2.75

PARTING THE HAIR

Part the hair for a Bob. Illustrations are on page 77.

Top parting: center, from the crown to the front.

Side parting: from ear-to-ear.

Front parting: triangle, from one-third of the top to the temples.

Back parting: triangle, from occipital bone to below the ears. Pin the upper section out of the way and smooth the rest of the hair down.

GUIDES

Back perimeter
Top of the nose   } OUTLINE
Temples
Eyebrows

Top-level checkpoint
Nose   } LAYERS
Top section
Sections and layers

ANGLES

Top: ninety-degree angle. *Fig. 2.76.*

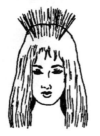

Fig. 2.76

Sides: 180 degree angle. *Fig. 2.77.*

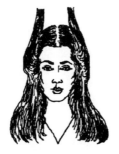

Fig. 2.77

Back: zero elevation. *Fig. 2.78.*

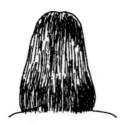

Fig. 2.78

LAYERED SECTIONS

Section thirteen corresponds to the top. *Fig. 2.79.*

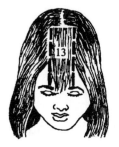

Fig. 2.79

Section fourteen, to the left side. *Fig. 2.80.*

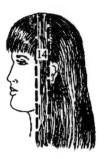

Fig. 2.80

Section fifteen, to the right side. *Fig. 2.81.*

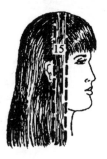

Fig. 2.81

CUTTING THE BOB

1. Cut a Bob as explained on page 76 and angle the sides as explained on page 62.

Once this step is completed return to this page and proceed to cut the top and side layers as follows:

CUTTING THE LAYERS

Section Thirteen: top

1. Re-establish ear-to-ear parting and pin the hair of the back out of your way to keep your parting clean.

2. Cut top-level checkpoint. See page 34 for details on how to cut this guide.

3. Stand next to the subject's left side.

4. Comb the top hair forward and make section thirteen, a two-inch wide section on top of the head from top-level checkpoint to the front.

5. Elevate section thirteen at a ninety-degree angle and center it using the nose as your guide.

6. Cut from top-level checkpoint to the front. Join those two points in a straight line. Do not cut into the checkpoint or the front outline, see that they drop uncut. Cut one-and-a-half to two inches at a time in small snips with the tips of the scissors. *Fig. 2.82.*

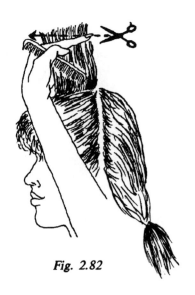

Fig. 2.82

Section Fourteen: left side

The sides have less hair. If the hair has been layered before you'll only need one section on the sides. However, if you find that the hair is very thick and long, make two sections. Do the upper section first and cut it at top-level length, then lift the lower section and cut it level with the first.

1. Stand next to the subject's left side.

2. Elevate the section at a 180 degree angle in a horizontal direction and drop the perimeter.

3. Cut it at top-level length. *Fig. 2.83.*

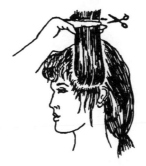

Fig. 2.83

If the length is very long you may need to over-extend the sides to avoid cutting the perimeter. *Fig. 2.84.* If you cut the perimeter while doing the layers you will change its shape and length. See page 131 for details on how to measure the hair to make sure the perimeter does not reach the guide.

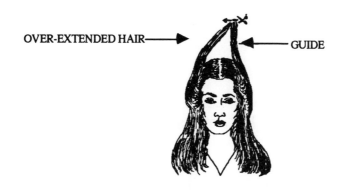

OVER-EXTENDED HAIR——▶   ◀—— GUIDE

Fig. 2.84

Section Fifteen: right side

1. Stand next to the subject's right side.

2. Lift the section at a 180 degree angle and drop the perimeter.

3. Cut horizontally at top-level length. *Fig. 2.85.*

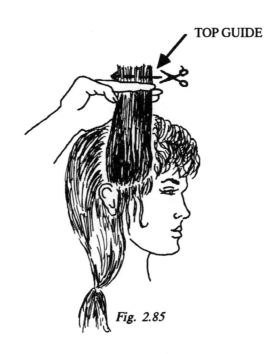

TOP GUIDE

Fig. 2.85

4. Comb the hair of the sides to the back. If she is satisfied with the length of the layers go on to check the haircut. If she is not, trim the side outline and shorten the layers.

CHECKING

Once you have cut the last section the next step is to check the haircut. If the sections are uneven, even them out. Do not make unnecessary cuts. Do not make new guides.

Ask yourself if you have made any of the following mistakes; they could be the reasons to uneven lengths of hair in your layers: Did you hold the hair at the correct angle? Did you follow the guide at all times? Did you part the hair correctly? Did you maintain the scissors straight with your fingers? Did you make clean partings?

1. Top: Stand behind the subject. Hold the hair at a ninety-degree angle and check the top in three horizontal sections. Start at top-level checkpoint and move towards the front. *Fig. 2.86.*

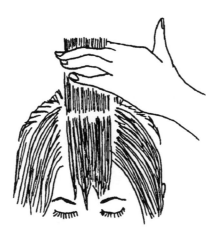

Fig. 2.86

2. Sides: Remain behind the subject. Re-adjust ear-to-ear parting. Elevate the sides at a 180 degree angle in a vertical direction and check that the line is straight with the top. *Fig. 2.87.*

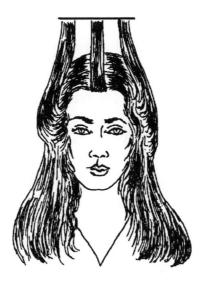

Fig. 2.87.

Now the haircut is completed. Breath deeply and smile.

REVIEW QUESTIONS

To ensure that you have learned the steps of the Bob variation, answer the following questions. The page numbers next to the questions indicate where the answers can be found.

1. How would you explain what one-length is? p. 30

2. What facial shapes look good with a Bob variation? pp. 43-46

3. How would you part the back of the hair to cut a Bob variation? p. 93

4. In what way is this haircut similar to the Bob? p. 93

5. In what way is this haircut similar to the long-layered? p. 93

6. What are the guides used to cut the back? p. 94

7. At what degrees of elevation would you hold the hair to cut the back, the top, and the sides? p. 94

8. How many layered sections are there? p. 95

9. Where would you start the haircut and where would you end it? pp. 96 and 98

10. What is the guide to the top length? p. 96

11. Why would you tie the hair of the back out of the way? p. 96

12. Is the hair of the sides cut in vertical or horizontal direction? p. 97

13. If the hair is very long, how would you make sure that you are not cutting the outline? p. 97

14. What is the guide to the side layers? p. 98

15. Briefly explain how would you check the top and back of this haircut? p. 99

F. BI-LEVEL WITH BOB BACK

The bi-level with Bob back is a combination of styles: the top and sides are cut in short layers as in a one-level; the back is one-length as in a Bob.

With the one-level top, bounce and volume are accomplished. The sides, short and close to the head, open up the face; the blunt cut in the back softens and frames the neck area. To change the looks of this style, for a sophisticated evening or a hot afternoon, you may pin up the back in a French twist or a Bun. *Fig. 2.88.*

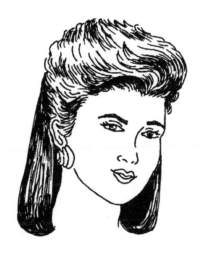

Fig. 2.88

PARTING THE HAIR

See illustrations of partings on Section D, page 77.

Top parting: center, from the crown to the forehead.

Side parting: from ear-to-ear.

Front parting: triangle, from one-third of the top to the temples.

Back parting: triangle, from the occipital bone to below the ears. Pin the upper section out of the way and smooth the rest of the hair down.

GUIDES

Back perimeter
Top of the nose   } OUTLINE
Temples
Eyebrows

Top-level checkpoint
Nose   } LAYERS
Top section
Sections and layers

ANGLES

Outline: zero elevation. *Fig. 2.89.*

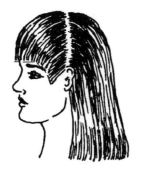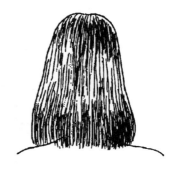

Fig. 2.89

Top and sides: ninety-degree angle. *Fig. 2.90.*

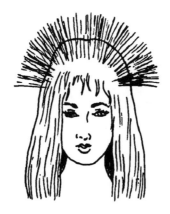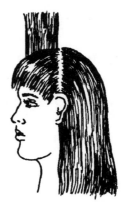

Fig. 2.90

LAYERED SECTIONS

Section seven corresponds to the top. *Fig. 2.91.*

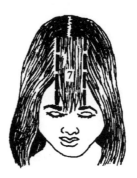

Fig. 2.91

Section eight, left side. *Fig. 2.92*

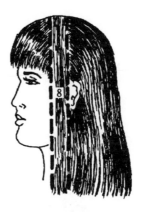

Fig. 2.92

Section nine, right side. *Fig. 2.93.*

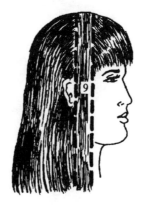

Fig. 2.93

CUTTING THE BACK

1. Cut a Bob in the back. See Section D, page 82-85 for details on how to cut a Bob back.

Once the back sections are completed return to this page and proceed to outline the front and the sides as follows:

TO OUTLINE THE FRONT

In this section of the outline act with care. As we mentioned before cowlicks and widow's peaks are common in the hairline.

a) From the Center to the Right Temple

1. Lift the subject's head straight.

2. Stand in front of the subject.

3. Re-adjust the triangle parting in the top.

4. Cut a center guide on top of the nose.

5. Cut from the top of the nose to below the temple. *Fig. 2.94.*

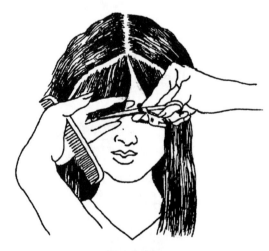

Fig. 2.94

Make sure the right side is even and get ready to cut the left side.

b) From the Center to the Left Temple

The left side of the front outline will be parted in two sections. This way you will always have your guide visible.

1. Cut section one and join it with the center guide. *Fig. 2.95.*

2. Cut section two from below the temple to section one and join them. Make sure you place your fingers in the same angle you had them on the other side. *Fig. 2.96.*

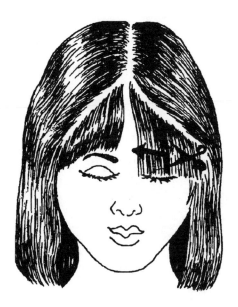

Fig. 2.95

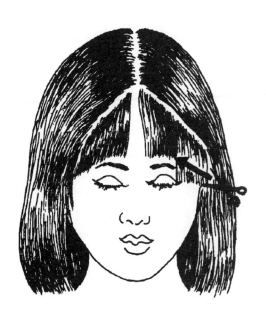

Fig. 2.96

3. Once the left side is finished stand back and observe. Do you have an even curvature? Is it too short, too long? If the hair is too long make a new guide in the center and start again. Adjustments should be made cutting one-quarter inch at a time. Remember that once the hair dries it will be shorter.

4. Breath deeply and get ready to cut the sides.

TO OUTLINE THE SIDES

a) Left Side

1. Re-establish ear-to-ear parting and pin up the hair of the back out of the way.

2. Stand next to the subject's left side.

3. Tilt the subject's head to the right side to have a clear view and a comfortable position to work.

4. Comb the hair down over the ear. *Fig. 2.97.*

5. Cut from the ear to the front the length agreed with the subject (top of the ear, mid-ear, or below the ear). Do not cut above the hairline. *Fig. 2.97.*

6. Comb the hair toward the front. *Fig. 2.98.*

7. Drop the outline. Cut in a upward direction toward the temple and meet the frontal outline. *Fig. 2.98.*

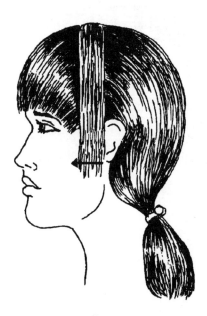

Fig. 2.97

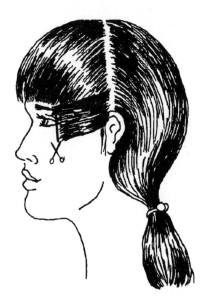

Fig. 2.98

Now the left side is finished. Make sure that the length is acceptable with the person and get ready to cut the right side.

b) Right Side

Once you are finished with the left side proceed to outline the right side using the same method.

1. Stand next to the subject's right side.

2. Re-adjust ear-to-ear parting.

3. Tilt the subject's head to the left side.

4. Comb the hair of the side over the ear. *Fig. 2.99.*

5. Cut from the front to the ear. *Fig. 2.99.*

6. Comb the hair towards the front. Fig. *2.100.*

7. Cut in a downward direction from below the temple to the cheek. *Fig. 2.100.*

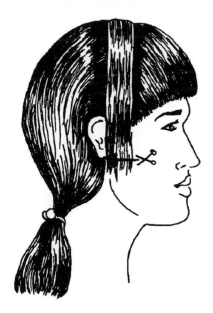

Fig. 2.99

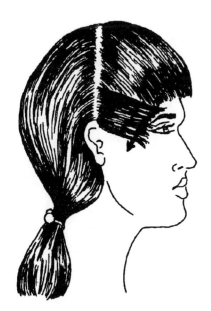

Fig. 2.100

Breath deeply; stand back and observe. You may use the bones of the ears as points of reference to make sure you have the same length on both sides.

Once the outline is complete start cutting layers on the top and side hair as follows:

CUTTING THE LAYERS

Section Seven: top

1. Re-establish ear-to-ear parting and keep the hair of the back pinned out of your way.

2. Cut top-level checkpoint. See Section F, page 34 for details on how to cut this guide.

3. Stand next to the subject's left side.

4. Comb the hair of the top forward and make a two-inch wide section from top-level checkpoint to the front.

5. Elevate it at a ninety-degree angle and cut from top-level checkpoint to the front. Join those two points in a straight line. Do not cut into the checkpoint or the front perimeter, see that they drop uncut. *Fig. 2.101.*

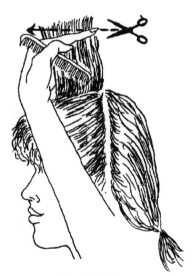

Fig. 2.101

Comb the top towards the back and make sure the length is acceptable. If it is too long trim the top layer. Adjustments should be made cutting one-quarter inch at a time.

Section Eight: left side

1. Remain next to the subject's left side.

2. Comb section seven forward and make a center parting on the top.

3. Re-adjust ear-to-ear parting and keep the hair of the back pinned out of your way.

4. Hold section eight at a ninety-degree angle in vertical direction.

5. Cut from the perimeter to the top. Join section eight to section seven. *Fig. 2.102.*

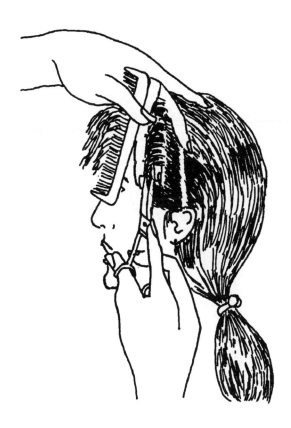

Fig. 2.102

Now the left side is completed. Comb the hair to the back and make sure that the length of the layers is acceptable. If it is not, trim the side outline and shorten the layers. Otherwise go on to the right side and cut it as follows:

Section Nine: right side

1. Stand behind the subject.

2. Elevate section nine at a ninety-degree angle. Make sure you are not pulling the section back towards you. If you do, it will be longer than section eight on the left side.

3. Cut from the perimeter to the top. Join section nine to section seven. See *Fig. 2.103.*

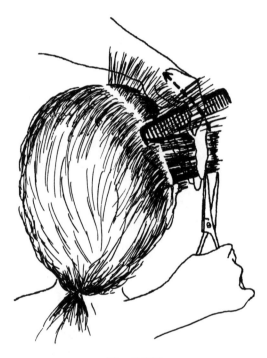

Fig. 2.103

CHECKING

Once you have cut the last section the next step is to check the haircut. If there are uneven sections, even them out. Do not make unnecessary cuts. Do not make new guides.

Ask yourself if you have made any of the following mistakes; they could be the reasons to uneven lengths of hair in your layers: Did you apply too much tension to some sections of hair? Did you follow the guide at all times? Did you make clean partings? Did you elevate the hair at the required angle?

Pin the hair of the back out of your way and stand behind the subject.

1. Top: Elevate the hair at a ninety-degree angle and check the top in three horizontal sections from the checkpoint to the front. *Fig. 2.104.*

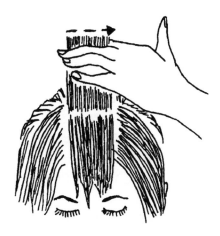

Fig. 2.104

2. Sides: Stand next to the subject to check the sides in horizontal sections at a ninety-degree angle. Start at the top and work your way down towards the hairline. *Fig. 2.105.*

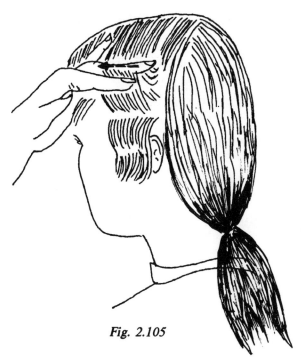

Fig. 2.105

Now the haircut is completed. Breath deeply and smile.

REVIEW QUESTIONS

To ensure that you have learned the steps to cut the bi-level with Bob back, answer the following questions. The page numbers next to the questions indicate where the answers can be found.

1. If the face was long, how could you cut this haircut to help correct the features. pg. 44

2. How is this haircut different to the Bob haircut? pg. 101

3. How is this haircut different to the one-level haircut? pg. 101

4. How would you part a bi-level with Bob back? pg. 101

5. List the guides used to cut the back. pg. 102

6. List the guides used to cut the top and sides. pg. 102

7. At what degree would you outline the hair? pg. 102

8. Would you elevate the hair to cut the back? pg. 102

9. At what degree of elevation would you layer the top and the sides? pg. 102

10. How many layered sections are there in this haircut? pg. 103

11. Explain the procedure to outline the sides. pp. 106-107

12. In what direction would you cut the sides? pg. 109

13. Where would you stand to layer the left side? the right side? pp. 109-110

14. Briefly explain how would you check this haircut. pg. 111

G. BI-LEVEL WITH LONG-LAYERED BACK

The bi-level combines two hairstyles: the one-level with short layers in the top and the sides, and the long-layered in the back.

This haircut is ideal for the person who enjoys the looks of short wavy hair around the face but does not want to lose their long hair in the back. By pinning up the hair this style offers different styling options, from the long look, to the short look. It is also a popular style among the men that prefer long hair with a tailored look. *Fig. 2.106.*

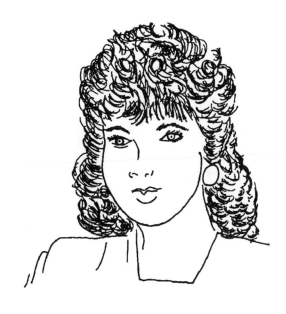

Fig. 2.106

PARTING THE HAIR

See illustrations of partings in Section A, page 51.

Top parting: center, from the crown to the forehead.

Side parting: from ear-to-ear.

Front parting: triangle, from one-third of the top to the temples.

Back parting: smooth it down with no partings.

GUIDES

Perimeter
Top of the nose
Temples
Eyebrows

} OUTLINE

Crown-level checkpoint
Nose
Top section
Sections and layers

} LAYERS

ANGLES

Top and sides: ninety-degree angle. *Fig. 2.107.*

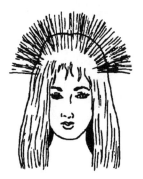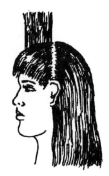

Fig. 2.107

Back: 180 degree angle. *Fig. 2.108.*

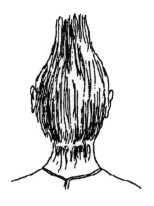

Fig. 2.108

LAYERED SECTIONS

Section one corresponds to the top. *Fig. 2.109.*

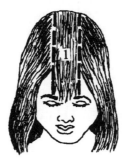

Fig. 2.109

Section two, left side. *Fig. 2.110.*

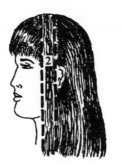

Fig. 2.110

Section three, right side. *Fig. 2.111.*

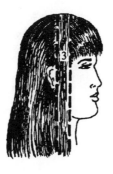

Fig. 2.111

115

Sections four and five, center of the back. *Fig. 2.112.*

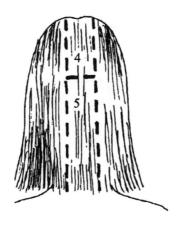

Fig. 2.112

Sections six and seven, left side of the back. *Fig. 2.113.*

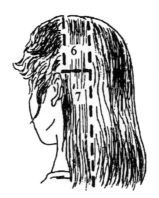

Fig. 2.113

Sections eight and nine, right side of the back. *Fig. 2.114.*

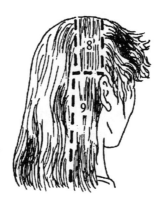

Fig. 2.114

OUTLINE

1. Outline the back, front, and sides. See Section B, page 53 for details on how to outline the hair.

Once the outline is completed return to this page and proceed to cut the layers as follows:

CUTTING THE LAYERS

Top: section one

1. Stand next to the subject's left side.

2. Cut crown-level checkpoint. See Section F, page 34 for details on how to cut this guide.

3. Comb the top hair forward.

4. Make a two-inch wide section, from crown-level checkpoint to the front.

5. Elevate section one at a ninety-degree angle and align it with the subject's nose.

6. Cut from the checkpoint to the front. Join those two points in a straight line. Do not cut into the checkpoint or the front perimeter, see that they drop uncut. *Fig. 2.115.*

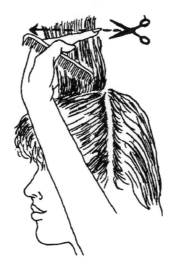

Fig. 2.115

Section Two: left side

1. Remain next to the subject's left side.

2. Make a center parting on the top.

3. Re-adjust ear-to-ear parting and pin the hair out of your way.

4. Cut section two from the perimeter to the top at a ninety-degree angle in a vertical direction. Use the perimeter as a guide to the length. *Fig. 2.116.*

5. Join section two to section one.

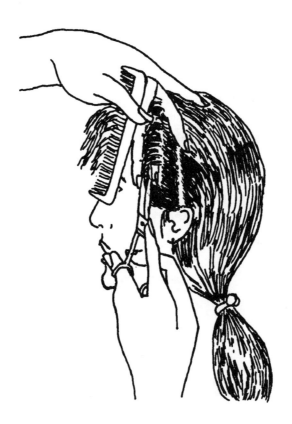

Fig. 2.116

Now the left side is completed. Comb the hair to the back and make sure that the length of the layers is acceptable with the person. If it is not, trim the side outline and shorten the layers. Otherwise cut the right side as follows:

Section Three: right side

1. Stand behind the subject's right shoulder.

2. Elevate section three at a ninety-degree angle.

3. Cut from the perimeter to the top in a vertical direction. Use the perimeter as a guide to the length. *Fig. 2.117.*

4. Join section three to section one.

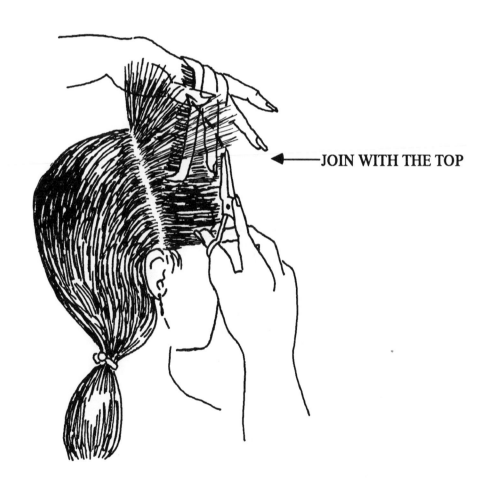

JOIN WITH THE TOP

Fig. 2.117

Now the sides are completed. Comb the hair and make sure both sides are equally long. Breath deeply and get ready to cut the back layers.

Sections Four Through Nine: back

When cutting the sections of the back under the occipital bone be careful with the perimeter. If the hair is very long you may need to over-extend the hair. If the hair does not reach the crown-level checkpoint when you lift it just drop it and move to the next section. See Section H, page 131 for more details.

1. Stand behind the subject. Comb the hair of the back down.

2. Make section four, a rectangular in the middle of the back, from the crown to the occipital bone.

3. Elevate section four at a 180 degree angle. *Fig. 2.118.*

4. Cut section four at crown-level checkpoint in a horizontal direction. See *Fig. 2.118.*

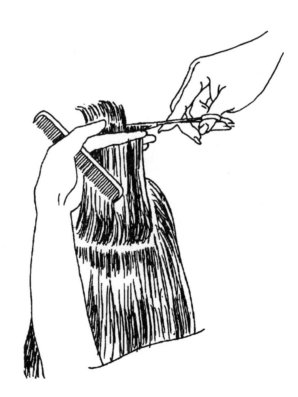

Fig. 2.118

5. Elevate section five at a 180 degree angle together with section four. Let the perimeter drop. Cut if there is hair extending over the crown-level checkpoint, otherwise drop the hair and continue to section six. *Fig. 2.119.*

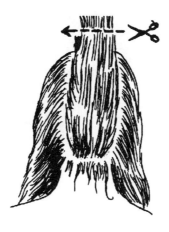

Fig 2.119

6. Make section six and include one-quarter inch of hair from section four as a guide to the length. *Fig. 2.120.*

7. Elevate and cut section six at a 180 degree angle. *Fig. 2.120.*

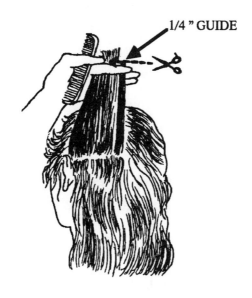

1/4 " GUIDE

Fig. 2.120

8. Elevate section seven at a 180 degree angle and cut it using section six as a guide. Cut if there is hair extending over section six. *Fig. 2.121.*

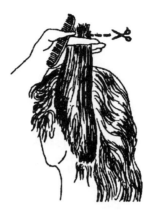

Fig. 2.121

9. Elevate section eight on the right side of the back and cut it at a 180 degree angle. Use section four as a guide to the length. *Fig. 2.122.*

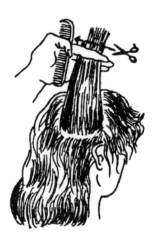

Fig. 2.122

10. Elevate section nine at a 180 degree angle together with section eight. Cut if there is hair extending beyond section eight. Otherwise drop the hair.

11. Breath deeply; comb the hair, and observe.

12. The layers are now completed. Get ready to check the haircut.

CHECKING

Check the haircut and even out the sections with crooked lines. Do not make unnecessary cuts. Do not make new guides.

Ask yourself if you made any of the following mistakes; they could be the reasons to uneven lengths of hair in your sections: Did you apply too much tension to some sections of hair? Did you follow the guide of previous sections at all times? Did you part the hair correctly? Did you place your hand in the appropriate angle? Did you consistently lift the hair at the required angle? Were some sections too big and others too small?

1. Crown: Stand behind the subject. Make a horizontal section at the crown. Elevate it at a 180 degree angle and even out if necessary. Ideally this section should be perfectly straight, if it is one-half inch longer on one side, it indicates that one side of the head has longer hair. If that's the case, start the haircut from the beginning. *Fig. 2.123.*

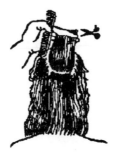

Fig. 2.123

2. Top: Stand behind the subject. Check the top in three horizontal sections from the crown to the front. Elevate the hair at a ninety-degree angle and if necessary even out the section. *Fig. 2.124.*

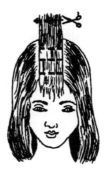

Fig. 2.124

3. Sides: Elevate the hair at a ninety-degree angle and check the sides in horizontal sections. *Fig. 2.125.*

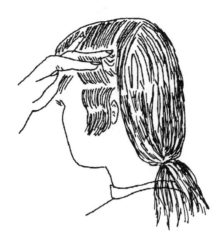

Fig. 2.125

4. Back: Elevate the hair at a 180 degree angle in vertical sections from the right side of the back to left side. *Fig. 2.126.*

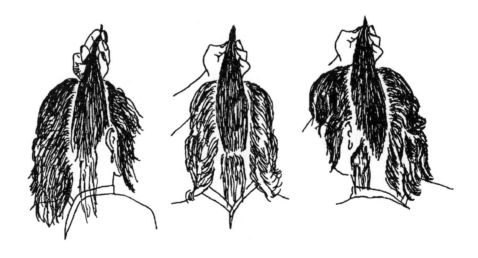

Fig. 2.126

Now the haircut is finished. Comb the hair and smile.

REVIEW QUESTIONS

To ensure that you have learned the steps to the bi-level with long-layered back, answer the following questions. The page numbers next to the questions indicate where the answers can be found.

1. In what way is this haircut similar to the one-level? p. 113

2. In what way is this haircut similar to the long-layered? p. 113

3. How would you part the hair? p. 113

4. At what angle would you cut the top and sides? p. 114

5. At what angle would you cut the back? p. 114

6. How many sections at the sides? p. 115

7. How many sections are there in the back? p. 116

8. In what direction would you cut the sides? p. 118

9. What are the guides to the top and side layers? pp. 117, 118

10. What would you do if the side layers are too long? p. 118

11. In what direction would you elevate and cut the hair of the back? p. 120

12. What would you do if the perimeter does not reach the top guide? pp. 120, 131

13. What are the guides to the back layers? pp. 120-122

14. How can you make sure that you are not cutting the perimeter? p. 120

15. Briefly explain how would you check this haircut. pp. 123-124

H. LONG-LAYERED

This haircut is perfect to give fullness and bounce to wavy, curly, and super-curly hair. It reduces hair bulk and yet maintains the length long. It is the style that offers the most sexy, sophisticated looks. *Fig. 2.127.*

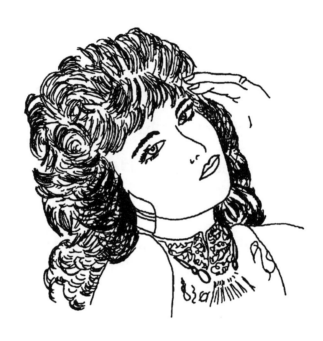

Fig. 2.127

PARTING THE HAIR

See illustrations of partings in Section A, page 51.

Top parting: center, from the crown to the forehead.

Side parting: from ear-to-ear.

Front parting: triangle, from one-third of the top to the temples.

Back: smooth it down with no partings.

GUIDES

Perimeter
Top of the nose   } OUTLINE
Temples
Eyebrows

Crown-level checkpoint
Nose
Top section   } LAYERS
Sections and layers

ANGLES

Top: ninety-degree angle. *Fig. 2.128.*

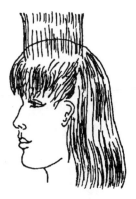

Fig. 2.128

Sides and back: 180 degree angle. *Fig. 2.129.*

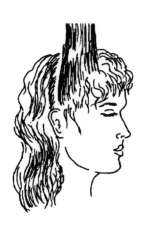
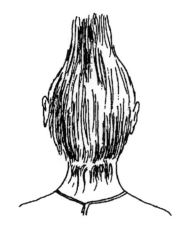

Fig. 2.129

127

LAYERED SECTIONS

Section one corresponds to the top. *Fig. 2.130.*

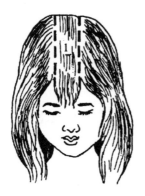

Fig. 2.130

Sections two and three, center of the back. *Fig. 2.131.*

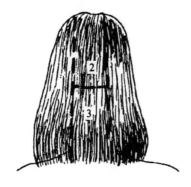

Fig. 2.131

Sections four and five, left side of the back. *Fig. 2.132.*

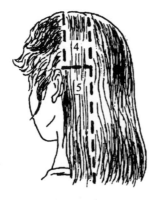

Fig. 2.132

Sections six and seven, right side of the back. *Fig. 2.133.*

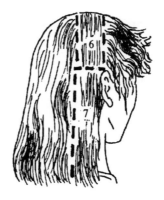

Fig. 2.133

Section eight, left side. *Fig. 2.134.*

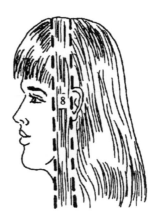

Fig. 2.134

Section nine, right side. *Fig. 2.135.*

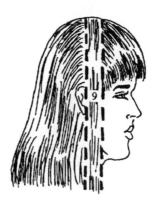

Fig. 2.135

OUTLINE

1. Outline the back, front, and sides. See Section B, page 53 for details on how to outline the hair.

Once the outline is completed return to this page and proceed to cut the layers as follows:

CUTTING THE LAYERS

1. Stand behind the subject.

2. Cut crown-level checkpoint. See Section F, page 34 for details on how to cut this guide.

Top: section one

1. Make section one, a two-inch wide parting on the top of the head.

2. Elevate section one at a ninety-degree angle.

3. Cut from the checkpoint to the front. *Fig. 2.136.*

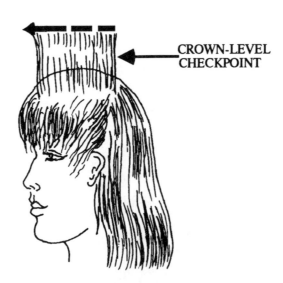

CROWN-LEVEL
CHECKPOINT

Fig. 2.136

Sections Two Through Seven: back

When the hair is elevated at a 180 degrees the outline has to drop. (If you cut the outline while giving layers you will change its length and shape.) In the beginning you may not be sure whether you are cutting the outline if the hair, being wet, sticks together as you elevate it. If you are afraid to miscalculate, cut the checkpoint, elevate a strand of hair from the hairline at 180 degree angle, and hold it at the ends. Elevate the checkpoint at a ninety-degree angle and measure. This way you will know if the perimeter extends beyond the checkpoint.

If the hair is very long you may find that the outline does not drop. In this case, you will need to over-extend the section to top-level checkpoint or further to make sure that the perimeter will not be cut. With experience you will know by looking at the length of the hair if it's necessary to over-extend the sections. *Fig. 2.137.*

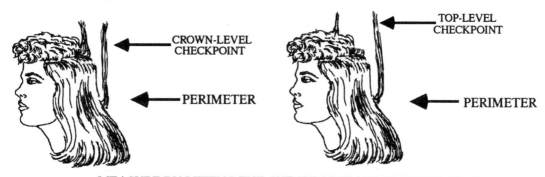

MEASURE BY LIFTING THE CHECKPOINT AND THE PERIMETER

Fig. 2.137

1. Stand behind the subject.

2. Make section two, a two-inch wide parting from the crown to the occipital bone.

3. Elevate section two at a 180 degree angle and cut it at checkpoint level in a horizontal direction. *Fig. 2.138.*

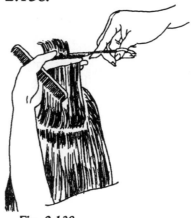

Fig. 2.138

4. Elevate section three at a 180 degree angle, allow the perimeter to drop. *Fig. 2.139.*

5. Cut the hair extending over the guide (section two). If the hair does not reach the guide just drop it and go on to the next section.

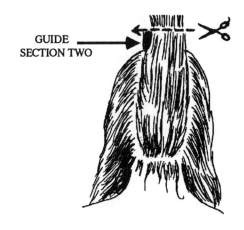

GUIDE
SECTION TWO

Fig. 2.139

6. Define section four in the left side of the back. Include one-quarter inch of section two as a guide to the length of section four.

7. Elevate and cut the hair at a 180 degree angle. *Fig. 2.140.*

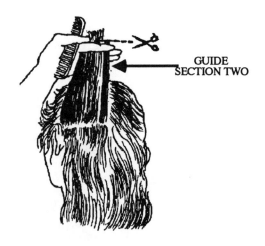

GUIDE
SECTION TWO

Fig. 2.140

8. Define section five from the occipital bone to the perimeter and elevate the section at a 180 degree angle.

9. Cut the hair extending over section four. *Fig. 2.141.*

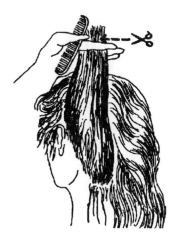

Fig. 2.141

10. Move to the right side of the back.

11. Lift and cut section six at a 180 degree angle. Include one-quarter inch of hair from section two as a guide to the length. *Fig. 2.142.*

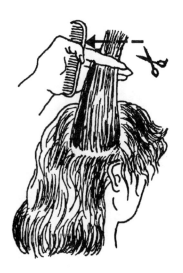

Fig. 2.142

133

12. Elevate section seven and repeat the same procedure. Use section six as a guide to the length. *Fig. 2.143*.

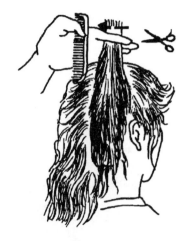

Fig. 2.143

Section Eight: left side

Usually the sides have less hair (especially if the hair has been layered before) so you'll only need one section at the sides. However, for very thick hair make two sections. If the hair is very long you may need to over-extend the hair. See page 97 for details.

1. Define section eight on the left side of the head.

2. Elevate it at a 180 degree angle and cut it level with section one on the top of the head. *Fig. 2.144*.

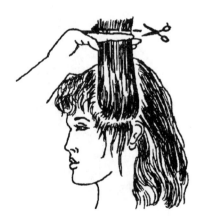

Fig. 2.144

Section Nine: right side

1. Repeat the procedure practiced on the left side to cut section nine. *Fig. 2.145.*

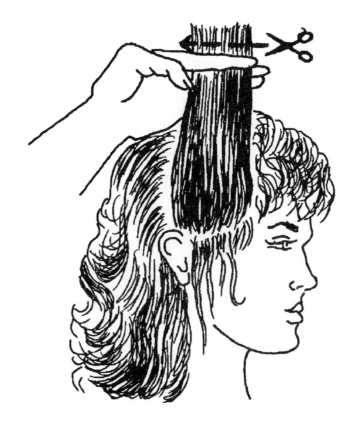

Fig. 2.145

2. Breath deeply and get ready to check the haircut.

CHECKING

When checking do not make unnecessary cuts or new guides. Even out the sections that are crooked or that have long wisps of hair.

Ask yourself if you made any of the following mistakes; they could be the reasons to uneven lengths of hair in your sections: Did you apply too much tension to some sections of hair? Did you follow the guide at all times? Did you part the hair correctly? Did some sections have more hair than others? Did you stretch the hair at the required angle?

1. Crown: Stand behind the subject. Elevate a horizontal section at the crown at a 180 degree angle and even it if necessary. Ideally it should be perfectly straight. If it is one-half inch or more longer on one side it indicates that one side of the head has longer hair. If that is the case start the haircut all over again. *Fig. 2.146.*

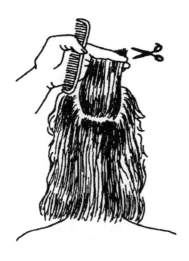

Fig. 2.146

2. Top: Stand behind the subject. Check the top at ninety-degree angle in three horizontal sections from the crown to the front. *Fig. 2.147.*

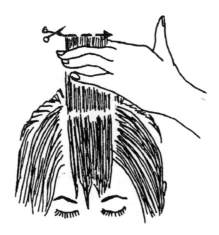

Fig. 2.147

3. Sides: Stand behind the subject. Elevate each side in vertical direction at a 180 degree angle. Make sure the line is straight with the top length. *Fig. 2.148*

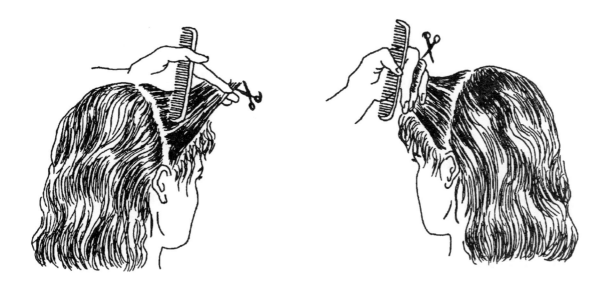

Fig. 2.148

4. Back: Starting at the right side of the back elevate the hair at a 180 degree angle in vertical sections. *Fig. 2.149.*

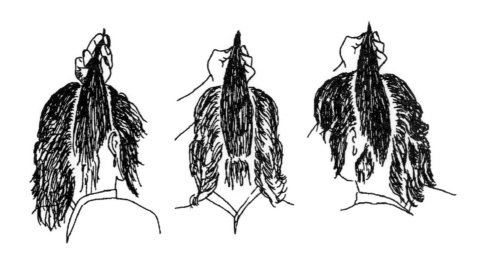

Fig. 2.149

REVIEW QUESTIONS

To ensure that you have learned the steps of the long-layered, answer the following questions. The page numbers next to the questions indicate where the answers can be found.

1. What does the crown-level checkpoint indicate? pg. 34

2. Is this a good haircut to reduce bulk? pg. 126

3. How is the hair parted? pg. 126

4. What is the degree of elevation at the top? pg. 127

5. What is the degree of elevation of the sides and the back? pg.127

6. If you are not sure that the perimeter is dropping how would you be able to tell that it does not reach the crown-level checkpoint? pg. 131

7. Why, in some cases, would the hair need to be over-extended? pg. 131

8. In what direction are the layers cut? pg. 131

9. Why would you elevate the sections under the occipital bone together with the upper sections? pg. 132

10. Section two serves as a guide to what other sections? pp. 133-134

11. Which are the guides to sections three, five, and seven? pp. 132-134

12. Which is the guide to sections nine and eight? pg. 135

13. In what direction would you check the hair? pp. 136-137

I. WEDGE

The Wedge is an all time favorite. It is an easy-care, comfortable coif with a feminine touch. In the Wedge the hair is graduated in reverse. The shortest point will be the back perimeter and the longest, the crown. There are many variations of the Wedge that together with the different textures and densities of the hair, will change the looks of this style. *Fig. 2.150.*

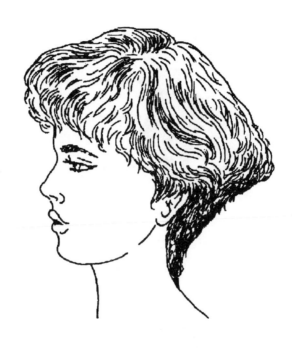

Fig. 2.150

PARTING THE HAIR

See illustrations of partings in Section A, page 51.

Top parting: center, from the crown to the forehead.

Side parting: from ear-to-ear.

Front parting: for bangs, triangle, from one-third of the top to the temples.

Back parting: V parting, from the top of the ears to the occipital bone. Pin the upper section out of the way and smooth the rest of the hair down.

GUIDES

Perimeter
Top of the nose   } OUTLINE
Temples
Eyebrows

Sections and layers } LAYERS

ANGLES

Back: zero elevation, forty-five-degree angle, and 180 degree angle. *Fig. 2.151.*

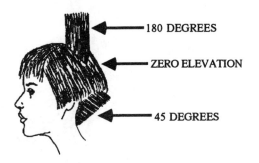

Fig. 2.151

Sides: forty-five-degree angle. *Fig. 2.152.*

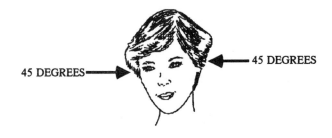

Fig. 2.152

Front: ninety-degree angle. *Fig. 2.153.*

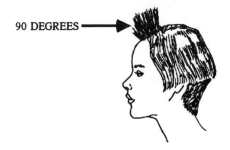

Fig. 2.153

LAYERED SECTIONS

The number of sections of the back may vary according to the size of the head, the width of the sections and the final look. Stop making sections when you reach the occipital bone. The sections should be approximately one-inch wide. In our sample haircut we will have eight sections in the back.

Sections one through eight, back. *Fig. 2.154.*

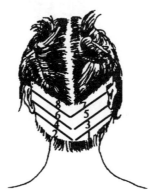

Fig. 2.154

Section nine, from crown to occipital bone. *Fig. 2.155.*

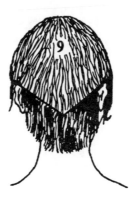

Fig. 2.155

Section ten, crown. *Fig. 2.156.*

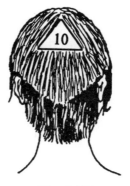

Fig. 2.156

141

Section eleven, left side. *Fig. 2.157.*

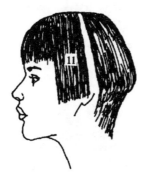

Fig. 2.157

Section twelve, right side. *Fig. 2.158.*

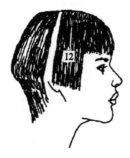

Fig. 2.158

Sections thirteen and fourteen, front. *Fig. 2.159.*

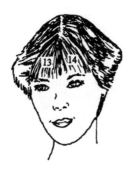

Fig. 2.159

OUTLINE

1. Outline the back, front, and sides. See Section B, page 53 for details on how to outline the hair.

Once the outline is completed return to this page and proceed to cut the layers as follows:

CUTTING THE LAYERS

Sections One Through Eight: back

1. Make the first section and pin up the rest of the hair out of the way.

2. Elevate the perimeter and section one at a forty-five-degree angle. *Fig. 2.160.*

3. Cut the section using the perimeter as a guide to the length. Do not cut into the perimeter, see that it drops uncut.

4. Cut horizontally from the right to the center in a downward direction to follow the contour of the head.

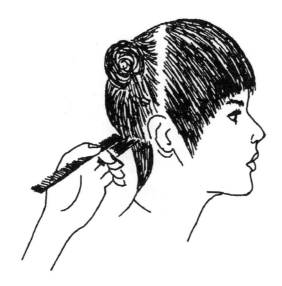

Fig. 2.160

5. Define section two.

6. Elevate it with the perimeter at a forty-five-degree angle. *Fig. 2.161.*

7. Cut from the center to the left in an upward direction. Use the perimeter and section one as your guides to length. In this way you'll be overlapping the sections for a blended effect in the layers.

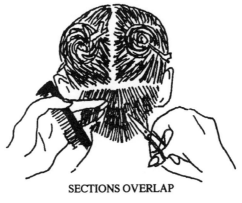

SECTIONS OVERLAP

Fig. 2.161

8. Bring down section three and four.

9. Pin up the rest of the hair out of the way.

10. Elevate section one and three at a forty-five-degree angle. Use section one as your guide. Make sure you do not cut section one but that it drops uncut. *Fig. 2.162.*

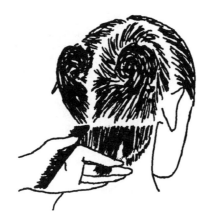

Fig. 2.162

11. Repeat the same steps with section four.

12. Continue the same procedure with each section until you reach the occipital bone.

Section Nine: back (from the crown to the occipital bone)

1. Once you have cut the last section, let the hair down and comb it. Starting at the right side, stretch the hair at zero elevation and cut toward the center, using section seven as a guide. *Fig. 2.163.*

2. Continue cutting from the center to the left ear. Use section eight as guide.

3. Do not cut the sections used as guides. If it is easier for you, elevate section nine to a forty-five-degree angle. This way you will be able to see the guide better and avoid cutting the previous sections.

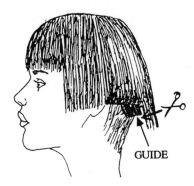

STRETCH THE HAIR AT 45º ANGLE OR AT ZERO ELEVATION

Fig. 2.163

Section Ten: crown

1. Make section ten, a triangle at the crown.

2. Lift the hair at a 180 degree angle. If there is a point cut it straight and drop the hair. This procedure will keep the hair from flipping up at the ends. *Fig. 2.164.*

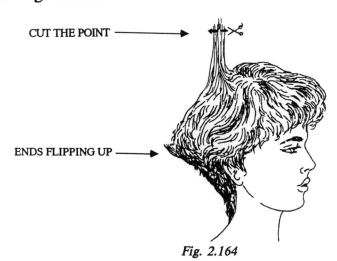

CUT THE POINT ⟶

ENDS FLIPPING UP ⟶

Fig. 2.164

Now the back is completed. Breath deeply and get ready to cut section eleven on the left side of the subject.

Section Eleven: left side

If the hair of the sides is very thick you may need to part it in half-horizontals. Cut the first layer at a forty-five-degree angle using the perimeter as your guide. Cut the second layer at a forty-five-degree angle using the length of the first layer as your guide. *Fig. 2.165.*

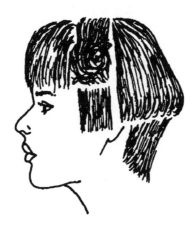

Fig. 2.165

1. Elevate the left side at a forty-five-degree angle in a horizontal direction. *Fig. 2.166.*

2. Use the perimeter as a guide to the length.

3. Allow the perimeter to drop.

4. Cut the left side in a horizontal direction from the ear to the front.

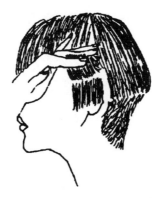

Fig. 2.166

Section Twelve: right side

1. Repeat the same procedure practiced on the left side to cut the right side.

You have now completed the sides. Breath deeply and get ready to cut the front as follows:

Sections Thirteen and Fourteen: front

1. Elevate the left side at a ninety-degree angle.

2. Drop the perimeter.

3. Cut the ends in a horizontal direction from the temple to the center. *Fig. 2.167.*

4. Repeat the procedure with the right side of the front. Cut the ends from the center to the temple. Now the front is slightly layered. For a more layered look see Chapter III, page 153.

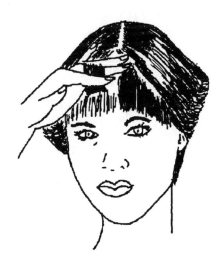

Fig. 2.167

You have now completed the front. Breath deeply, comb the hair, observe, and get ready to check the haircut.

CHECKING

Ask yourself if you made any of the following mistakes; they could be the reasons to uneven lengths of hair in your sections: Did you apply too much tension to some sections of hair? Did you follow the guide at all times? Did you part the hair correctly? Did some sections have more hair than others? Did you place your hand in the appropriate angle? Did you stretch the hair at the required angle? Did you cut into the guide?

When checking do not make unnecessary cuts or new guides, simply even out the sections that are slightly crooked.

1. Back: Elevate the back at forty-five-degrees in vertical sections. Move from the center to the right and from the center to the left. The hair must be increasingly longer from the hairline to the occipital bone. *Fig. 2.168.*

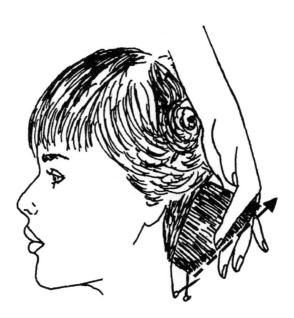

Fig. 2.168

2. Sides: Elevate the hair at forty-five-degrees from the ear to the front in vertical sections. The hair must be increasingly longer from the perimeter to above the ears. *Fig. 2.169.*

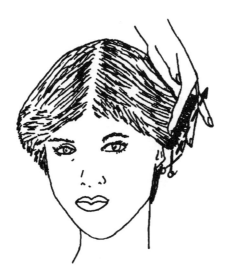

Fig. 2.169

3. Front: Check in vertical sections at a forty-five-degree angle. Move from the center to the right side and from the center to the left side. *Fig. 2.170.*

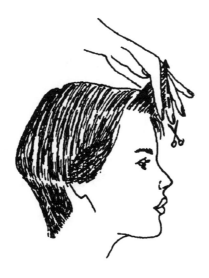

Fig. 2.170

REVIEW QUESTIONS

To ensure that you have learned the steps of the Wedge, answer the following questions. The page numbers next to the questions indicate where the answers can be found.

1. How short should the length of this haircut be? p. 53

2. Where is the shortest and the longest hair? p. 139

3. How should the Wedge be parted? p. 139

4. At what degree-angle would you elevate the hair to cut a Wedge? p. 140

5. What are the guides to cut the outline? p. 140

6. How many sections are there in the back, sides, and front? pp. 141-142

7 Which is the initial guide to the length of the back? p. 143

8. Are the layers cut in a vertical or horizontal direction? p. 143

9. List other guides to the sections of the back? p. 144

10. Why is there a section on the crown? p. 145

11. At what point should you stop making layers in the back? p. 145

12. If the hair is thick how would you part the sides? p. 146

13. How would you layer the sides and the front? pp. 146, 147

14. How would you check the back? pp. 148-149

15. How would you check the front and sides? p. 149

16. In what direction would you hold the hair to check it? p. 149

Chapter III

MORE TECHNIQUE

Once you have practiced the basic haircuts explained in Chapter II, you will be prepared to learn techniques to give accent to the haircuts. With these easy techniques you can emphasize movement of the hair in one direction; give volume to the top; frame the face; give extra layers to the front and character to the back.

Read through the different techniques and practice them later.

How to Cut Wisps of Hair

A few strands of hair in the front or in the sideburns area give softness and are flattering to the face. However if the wisps are too short, the cowlicks in the hairline area will make them curl and stick up.

Cut the wisps semi-dry; also cut the guide below the eyebrows, stretching the hair without tension.

1. Ask the person how much hair she likes to have covering her forehead. The more hair you take, the more the wisps will resemble bangs.

2. Cut a strand of hair above the nose. This will be your guide.

3. Hold all the hair selected in the center of the forehead.

4. Slide your fingers to the end of the guide and when the guide snaps released, cut above the fingers. *Fig. 3.1.*

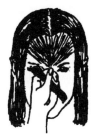

Fig. 3.1

To give sideburns wisps, bring down a few strands of hairline hair, and cut them no shorter than the length of the ear. *Fig. 3.2.* Comb the hair towards the cheek and shape it. *Fig. 3.3*

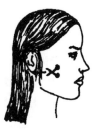

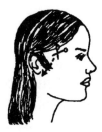

Fig. 3.2   *Fig. 3.3*

How to Layer Bangs

Bangs can sometimes have a very heavy and thick appearance. To make them lighter and give them a layered look, proceed as follows:

1. Make a triangle parting from one-third of the top to the temples.

2. Elevate the section at a ninety-degree angle in a vertical direction. *Fig. 3.4*

3. Allow the outline to drop.

4. Cut the ends of the hair at a ninety-degree angle. *Fig. 3.5.*

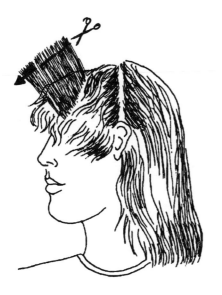

Fig. 3.4

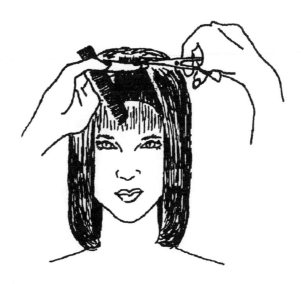

Fig. 3.5

5. Elevate the bangs again; this time in a horizontal position and trim any uneven ends.

How to Spike the Hair of the Top

The hair can be layered or it can be one-length. To spike the top proceed as follows:

1. Make triangle parting from crown-level checkpoint to the temples. (To give less dramatic spikes use the top-level checkpoint.)

2. Make crown-level checkpoint.

3. Elevate the section at a ninety-degree angle.

4. Cut the hair from crown-level checkpoint to the front about two inches long. *Fig. 3.6.*

5. With thinning shears, cut the same section an inch away from the scalp. This procedure will remove weight and the shorter ends will give lift to the longer hair.

6. Cut with thinning shears only two times.

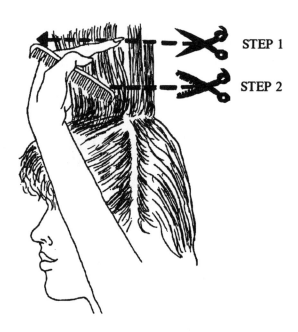

STEP 1

STEP 2

Fig. 3.6

7. To keep the spiked hair sticking up, style it with mousse, gel, hair spray, or setting lotion.

How to Cut the Top for Forward Motion

If you want the top to move forward, the crown hair needs to be longer than the front hair. Cut it as follows:

1. Cut the outline.

2. Cut crown-level checkpoint if the hair is layered, or top-level checkpoint if the haircut has a bob back.

3. Make a triangular parting from the checkpoint to the front.

4. Elevate the hair at a ninety-degree angle and place your fingers downward to give less length to the front. *Fig. 3.7.*

5. Cut from checkpoint to the front. Make sure the outline drops uncut.

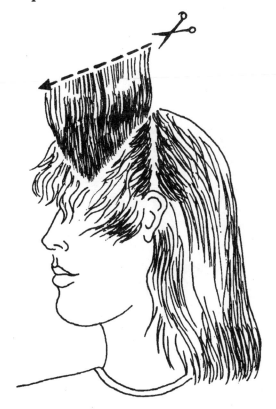

Fig. 3.7

6. If the hair is too thick in front, elevate one-third of the front hair and cut it twice with thinning shears. Keep a distance of two inches from the scalp. Remember to drop the outline and avoid thinning out the hairline hair.

155

How to Cut the Top for Backward Motion

If you want the top hair to move backwards, you need the front hair to be longer than the crown hair. Cut it as follows:

1. Cut the outline.

2. Cut crown-level checkpoint if the hair is layered, or top-level checkpoint if the haircut has a bob back.

3. Make a triangular parting from the checkpoint to the front.

4. Elevate the hair at a ninety-degree angle and place your fingers in an upward direction to give length to the front.

5. Cut from the checkpoint to the front. *Fig. 3.8.*

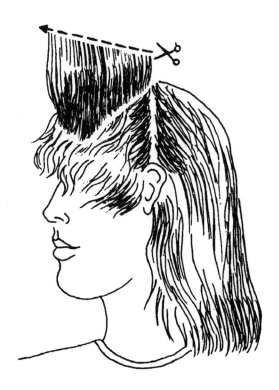

Fig. 3.8

How to Cut Ducktails

To give Ducktails, the hair at the center of the back needs to be the shortest point. The sections of hair have to slightly increase in length as they get closer to the back of the ears.

1. Shape the outline.

2. Make a quarter-inch section in the center of the back and cut it to make a guide. Do not cut into the outline, make sure its shape is maintained.

3. Make vertical sections moving from the center to the back of the ears, and cut them at a forty-five degree angle. *Fig. 3.9*

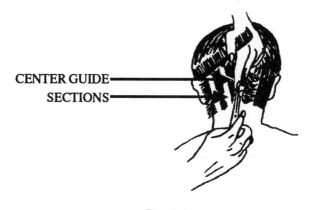

CENTER GUIDE
SECTIONS

Fig. 3.9

If you have completed a one-level haircut and the subject wants the look of Ducktails, gather the hair of the back in the center and elevate it at a ninety-degree angle. Cut from the perimeter to the occipital bone. *Fig. 3.10.*

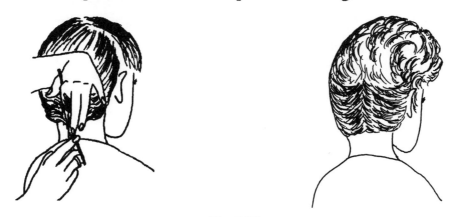

Fig. 3.10

Make sure to style the hair of the back towards the center, and show the person how to comb the hair to accomplish the desired look.

How to Blow-Style the Hair

Once you have finished a haircut, you can proceed to blow-dry the hair to mold it into the look you want. Before starting the blow-drying make sure the hair is evenly damp. If it is wet, be sure to towel dry it first. Remember that when you apply heat to wet, stretched hair, it will contract and cause breakage. On damp hair, you can apply mousse, gel or a hair protecting lotion to prepare the hair for drying.

Choose the appropriate brush for the length and type of hair you are going to dry. There are half-round brushes of different sizes, good for rolling motions. A brush that allows the air to pass through for quick drying, is the vent brush. Radial brushes are great to style the Bob and Bob variations. The small radial brushes are useful to give direction and volume to one-level and bi-level haircuts, as well as layered tops and sides. Keep in mind that more people today want a natural finish which will not require forcing the hair in place by overheating it.

To dry super-curly hair, use a light conditioner worked in damp hair, then retouch the hair with the curling iron, and apply hair spray to maintain the shape. If you want to keep the hair in place without the hard finish of hair spray, use mousse before blow-drying the hair. Always aim the air downwards, from the roots to the ends, or use a diffuser to give a curly finish with no fly-away hair.

Blow-dry the roots first to give the style volume and direction, then do the ends. Keep the blow-dryer at least six inches away to avoid burning the scalp or the hair, and watch out for the ears, they often get burned. Divide the hair in sections to keep the drying organized. Do not roll thick sections of hair, instead roll sections approximately two inches wide if the hair is short. If the hair is long, the sections will need to be smaller. If you take small sections you will do a better job and finish faster. For quick blow-drying try the following technique:

1. Part the hair of the back in the middle. With a radial brush dry the base of the hair. Then start drying it in sections from the center to behind the ears on either side of the back. *Fig. 3.11.*

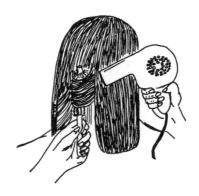

Fig. 3.11

2. Next, blow-dry the sides. *Fig. 3.12*

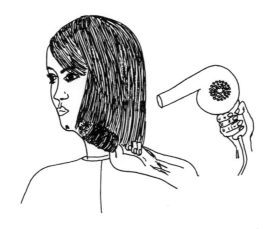

DRYING THE SIDES

Fig. 3.12

3. Finally, do the top following the natural direction of the hair. *Fig. 3.13.*

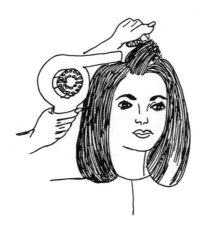

DRYING THE TOP

Fig. 3.13

For a sleek look, roll the hair of the back in small sections with the curling iron. To make sure that you don't burn the hair, place a finger on the hair that has been rolled, count to ten and release the hair. If you feel your finger getting too hot before you get to ten, release the hair immediately. Let the curl cool before brushing.

For extra volume, apply mousse to towel dried hair, tilt the head down and dry it with a vent brush or fingers. Throw the hair back and arrange it with a hair pick. To create more volume, tease the hair in the areas desired, and apply hair spray while lifting the hair with a pick.

Another method of giving more lift to the top and sides is by applying gel to the roots of the hair and drying them with a vent brush. When the hair has been completely blow-styled lift the hair with a hair pick and apply a spritz of hair spray to the roots to maintain the lift.

For contour, apply mousse and blow-dry the hair in small sections with a radial brush appropriate to the length of the hair.

For a more natural, casual look, blow-dry the hair between your fingers holding it straight out to give it lift.

Finally, for lots of curls, try scrunch drying. Squeeze the hair in a fist and allow the air to circulate through your fingers. When each section is dry, switch the dryer to a cool setting to fix the curl. Scrunch drying works well with the diffuser. *Fig. 3.14*

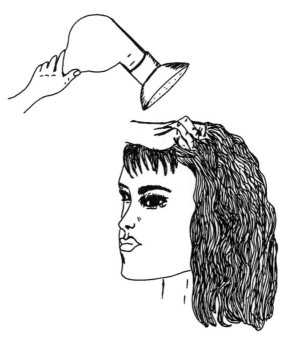

SCRUNCH DRYING

Fig. 3.14

Chapter IV

CLIPPER CUTTING TECHNIQUES

If you want to to cut short layers, flat-tops, sideburns, mustaches, and beards with speed and accuracy, learn to handle the clippers well. In this chapter you will learn 1) the different types of clippers and their functions, 2) what techniques to use when cutting with clippers, 3) how to cut some of the most popular hairstyles. After studying this chapter, all your fears about cutting with clippers should disappear.

Before starting, be sure to select the best-suited clipper for the style you will be creating. If a particular style requires hair sculpturing, buy clippers with interchangeable blades. This type of clipper usually includes five different sets of blades selected for cutting form lines, sculpturing, tapering, thinning and removing bulk. If additional blade sets are needed, they may be obtained from the distributor in a wide range of sizes. *Fig. 4. 1.*

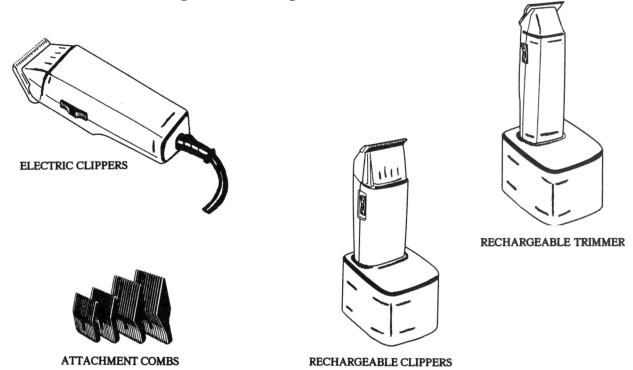

ELECTRIC CLIPPERS

RECHARGEABLE TRIMMER

ATTACHMENT COMBS

RECHARGEABLE CLIPPERS

DIFFERENT TYPES OF CLIPPERS AND ATTACHMENT COMBS

Fig. 4.1

Clippers are also available with attachment combs that may be used with interchangeable or fixed blades. The attachment combs are snapped over the blade to separate it from the scalp and give the hair different lengths. These combs are usually numbered "1" through "4" depending on the desired hair length. Attachment Number One leaves the hair approximately 1/8" long; No. Two, 1/4" long; No. Three, 3/8" long; and No. Four, 1/2" long. *Fig. 4.1, 4.2.* Using these combs will help you cut the hair faster and with greater accuracy. In addition, some clippers have a blade lever to adjust the blade to two or more settings. The blade lever opens or closes the blade. When the blade is closed, the teeth are even, and less tapering is accomplished; when open, the two layers of teeth in the blade are separated, and more taper is accomplished.

Clippers may be electric, rechargeable or both. The rechargeable clipper is cordless and lightweight; it brings snap-on combs or stainless steel blade sets for closer cutting. If rechargeable, they include a stand-up charger which may have an indicator light to show when the clipper is being charged.

The rechargeable trimmer is slimmer than the clippers, and better suited for light trimming, final touch-ups and sensitive areas. Trimmers are available in different sizes; the larger ones are excellent for entire cuts and more comfortable to hold than the clippers if you have small hands. Some of the trimmers bring snap-on combs and stainless steel blade sets, for closer cutting and texturizing. Rechargeable clippers and trimmers give you complete freedom of movement and may be used without electrical power; however in time the batteries will have to be replaced and this may be a costly inconvenience.

Choose clippers with ice-tempered, stainless steel blades; they will last longer. Give good care to your clippers; with just a bit of cleaning and a drop of clipper oil in the blades before and after each haircut, you will keep them in good operating condition for many years. Beware not to sanitize them with wet solutions; if you should touch the coil of wet clippers when these are plugged into an electrical outlet, you could suffer an electric shock. Always unplug them before cleaning and read the safety and care instructions before using them for the first time. The instructions also bring information on how to align, adjust, and clean the blades.

For beginners, clippers with attachment combs should be sufficient. Later on, after experimenting with them, it will be easier to decide if a better, more versatile type of clipper is needed.

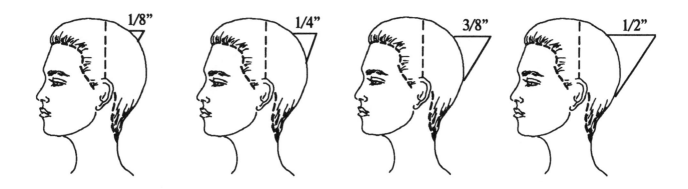

HAIR LENGTHS OBTAINABLE WHEN USING THE ATTACHMENT COMBS

Fig. 4.2

163

TECHNIQUES

There are several techniques for cutting with clippers; each will be explained with an example. After practice, you will know how to cut with each technique, and which to choose when cutting the different styles. The techniques are: a) freehand, b) clippers-over-fingers, and c) clippers-over-comb.

For further instruction, refer to the appendix of this book for information about the videotape *Haircutting With Clippers,* which shows, in action, how to use the three techniques described below.

a) Freehand Technique

The freehand technique is utilized to cut the hair, beard, mustache, and around the ears. With this technique you will not use the comb or fingers to guide you; instead the clippers will be placed directly on the scalp or face.

<u>How to cut the beard and mustache</u>

If the beard and mustache are short, they should be trimmed once a week, if long, up to once a month.

1. Discuss with the individual how long he wants his beard and choose the attachment according to the desired length, long, medium or short.
2. Comb the section to be cut.
3. Place the clippers flat on his face at the bottom hairline, and slide them upward against the direction of the hair growth. *Fig. 4.3.*

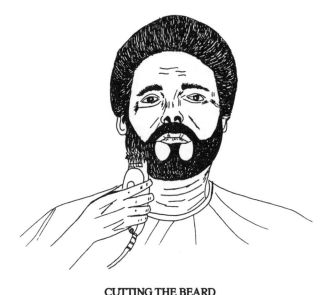

CUTTING THE BEARD
Fig. 4.3

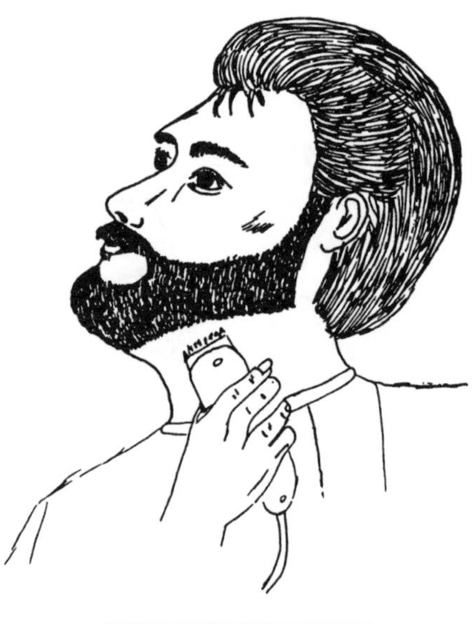

OUTLINING THE BEARD
Fig 4.4

4. Comb the hair down and cut over the same section more than once to be sure you don't miss any strands of hair.

5. Continue in an orderly fashion from one side of the face to the other. Comb with one hand and cut with the other until all sections are cut.

6. Even out the outline of the beard with the trimmer. Try to follow its natural line and cut any hair that stands out from the ears, neck and face. *Fig. 4.4.*

7. To cut the length of the mustache, place the trimmer above the lip and move it slowly supporting your hand with the comb, your free hand or the person's face. If your hand should slip while cutting, you can ruin a perfect mustache. *Fig. 4.5.* To thin the mustache, place the comb through the hair and cut the exceeding hair. *Fig. 4.6.*

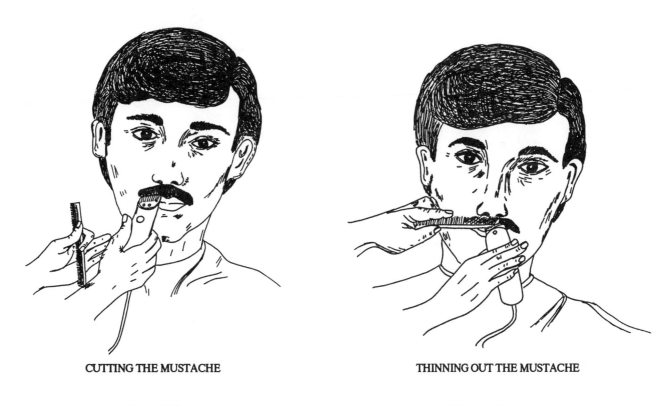

CUTTING THE MUSTACHE

Fig. 4.5

THINNING OUT THE MUSTACHE

Fig. 4.6

Now the mustache and beard are finished. Comb the hair down and check if you missed any strands of hair. Also check if the outline of the mustache is straight. If not, make the necessary adjustments.

165

b) Clippers-Over-Fingers Technique

To use this technique, you must pick up the hair with the comb and hold it between your fingers, just as you do when using the scissors. Also you will have to switch the comb from one hand to the other; all this is done while holding the clippers with your dominant hand. *Fig. 4.7.* This procedure is difficult at first, especially if you have small hands and are using heavy clippers.

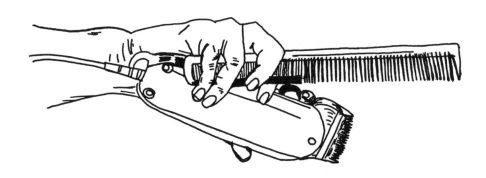

HAND POSITION, CLIPPER OVER FINGERS TECHNIQUE

Fig. 4.7

The long-layered may be cut with a symmetrical or an asymmetrical look. Both styles will be explained. *Fig. 4.8.*

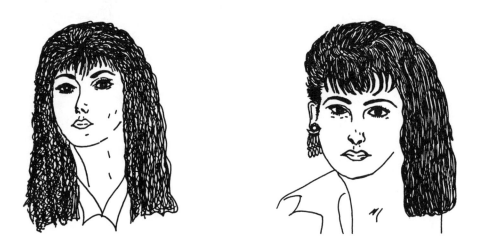

SYMETRICAL AND ASSYMETRICAL LONG LAYERED

Fig. 4.8

Long-Layered

1. Damp the hair and comb it free of tangles.

2. Outline the sections of hair indicated on pages 53-61, and use the clippers as shown below. *Fig. 4.9.*

3. Be sure to cut each section of hair in two steps. First, slide the corner of the clippers over the fingers; and second, even out the same section pressing the clippers onto the fingers. *Fig. 4.9.*

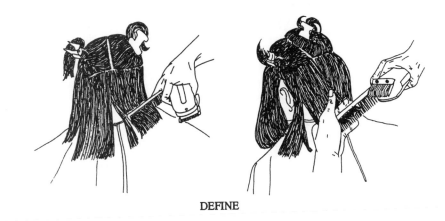

DEFINE

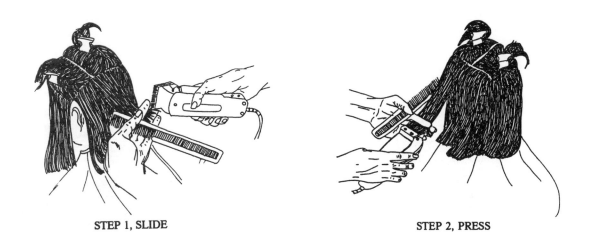

STEP 1, SLIDE   STEP 2, PRESS

CUTTING AN OUTLINE

Fig. 4.9

Once you have finished the outline, cut the checkpoint and the layered sections as shown in the long-layered haircut described on page 126. Be sure to cut the layers with the "sliding and pressing" procedure shown in *fig. 4.9.*

If you wish the asymmetrical look, so popular these days, you may cut one side shorter after you have finished cutting the layers. To do the asymmetrical look, follow these directions:

1. Find the natural part as described in page 41. Once the natural part has been determined, choose the side with less hair and cut it shorter. Leave the hair parted while cutting the side. *Fig. 4.10.*

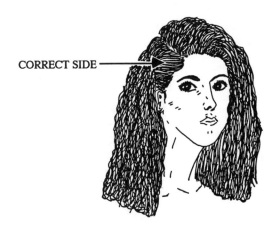

CORRECT SIDE

Fig. 4.10

2. Make a side section, comb the section forward and outline it. *Fig. 4.11.*

3. Comb the section down and outline it in a horizontal direction. *Fig. 4.12.*

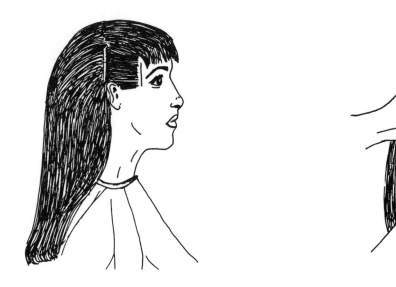

SIDE PARTING AND OUTLINING

Fig. 4.11   *Fig. 4.12*

4. If the person wants one side very short and close to the scalp, cut the outline above the ear and then proceed to cut with the clippers after placing the correct attachment. *Fig. 4.13.*

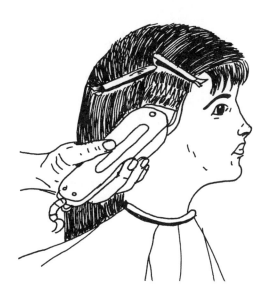

LAYERING WITH CLIPPERS AND ATTACHMENT COMB

Fig. 4.13

5. If a longer less dramatic look is preferred, cut the outline at mid-ear and use the clippers-over-fingers technique to cut the layers. *Fig. 4.14.* Comb the section down and layer it from the outline to the top in a vertical direction. *Fig. 4.14.*

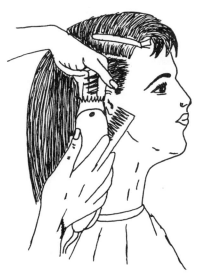

LAYERING WITH THE FINGERS

Fig. 4.14

6. Check the hair in horizontal sections from the outline to the top. *Fig. 4.15.*

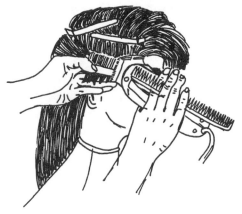

CHECKING THE SECTION

Fig. 4.15

Now the haircut is finished. Comb the hair and check if there are any sections that need more trimming.

c) Clippers-Over-Comb Technique

Men's hair, *fig. 4.16,* is easily tapered with the clippers-over-comb technique. The clippers, without attachments, are held with the dominant hand, and the comb with the opposite hand. The comb will elevate the hair and determine how much hair should be cut; the clippers are slid over the teeth, and any exceeding hair, is cut. This technique is fast and easy, especially to cut straight or wavy hair. When cutting super-curly hair, the comb should not be rotated; it should be held at the angle desired while you cut any hair exceeding the comb.

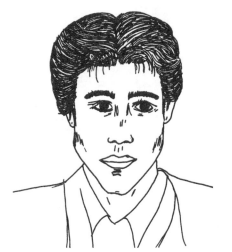

MEN'S HAIR

Fig. 4.16

How to Taper Men's Hair

1. Damp the hair.

2. Outline the hair following the same procedure described for the clippers-over-finger technique on page 53.

3. Once the hair has been outlined, start tapering in the back center section.

4. With the comb in a horizontal position, lift the hair at a forty-five-degree angle. With your dominant hand, place the clippers over the comb, and gently slide them over the teeth. Cut all the hair that exceeds the comb. Be sure to place the comb at the same angle and at the same distance from the head each time. *Fig. 4.17.*

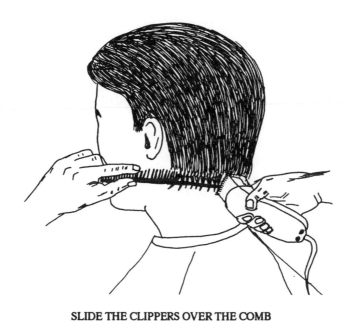

SLIDE THE CLIPPERS OVER THE COMB

Fig. 4.17

5. Once the back sections are finished, repeat the procedure on the sides, starting at the hairline and moving upward.

6. To cut the top, hold the comb in a horizontal position and pick up the crown hair at a ninety-degree angle.

7. Lift the hair in small sections and cut towards the front. *Fig. 4.18.*

171

8. With the trimmer, shape the sideburns and retouch the neckline. *Fig. 4.19.*

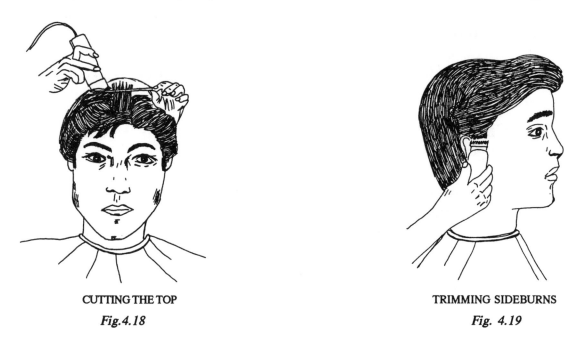

CUTTING THE TOP

Fig.4.18

TRIMMING SIDEBURNS

Fig. 4.19

Once the haircut is finished, comb the hair and check if some sections are heavier or longer. Make the necessary adjustments.

How to Cut a Flattop

To cut the Flattop *(fig. 4.20)* the freehand and clippers-over-comb techniques are used. The Flattop may be cut with many variations; the hair may be cut with attachments No. 3 or No. 4, or the front may be left longer and combed towards the back.

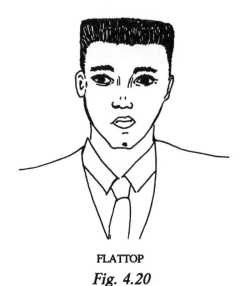

FLATTOP

Fig. 4.20

When cutting super-curly hair be sure to untangle it first, picking the hair up and away from the scalp with a pick. When the hair is straight, damp the hair, apply gel, and blow-dry the top hair straight up.

1. Select the appropriate attachment. If the hair is wanted very short and close to the scalp, choose attachment No. 1; if longer, No. 2. Be sure to determine the length desired before starting to cut.

2. Start at the hairline, place the clippers flat on the head and slide them straight up. *Fig. 4.21.*

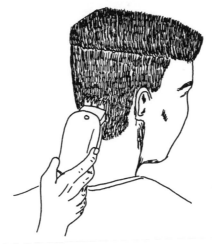

PLACE CLIPPERS FLAT ON THE HEAD

Fig. 4.21

3. Comb the hair down and cut over the same section more than once to be sure you don't miss any hair. Do not round the sides.

4. Be sure the cowlick area is cut short. *Fig. 4.22.*

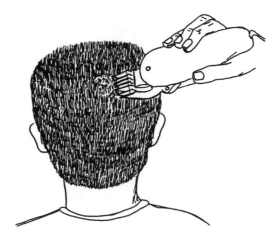

CUT THE COWLICK SHORT

Fig. 4.22

173

5. To cut the top, remove the attachment; hold the comb in a horizontal position and pick up the top hair at a ninety-degree angle.

6. Lift the hair in small sections and cut towards the front. *Fig. 4.23.*

7. To check for any hair you may have missed, lift the hair in small sections from the front to the back.

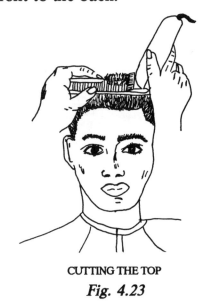

CUTTING THE TOP

Fig. 4.23

8. Place the comb in a vertical position and shape the sides of the top moving from back to front. *Fig. 4.24.*

9. With the trimmer retouch the sideburns and neckline hair.

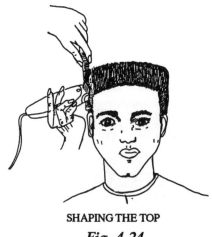

SHAPING THE TOP

Fig. 4.24

Now the Flattop is finished. Check for any hair that stands out and make the necessary adjustments. When using the clippers without a comb or attachment, your hand will have no support or guide. Be careful; it can very easily move and cut the hair too short.

Chapter V

ANALYZING THE HAIR

Healthy hair is beautiful hair. This is a simple statement, yet difficult to grasp; for most people, impatient and unfamiliar with treatments and procedures to improve their hair, will try to hide the damage with harsh chemical processes. Yes, it is possible to enjoy the hair color you like so much, or the permanent wave you've just got to have, but remember, they will only look beautiful if the hair is healthy.

In Chapter I we discussed the hair and how it is affected by chemicals, weather, illness, and many other factors. It is important to know and understand how and why the hair is changed by internal and external forces, and to learn to analyze the hair. Only then, you will know how to maintain its health and natural beauty.

A hair analysis is necessary to determine if the hair is really damaged and the extent of that damage. It consists of three steps, 1) scalp inspection, 2) hair test, and 3) questions. This analysis only takes a few minutes and will help you recommend the changes, products, and treatments to improve the condition of the hair.

Begin the analysis with an inspection of the scalp for irritations, scabs, redness or anything unusual. Take a special look for signs of pediculosis or head lice. Lice are small grayish-tan wingless insects; the eggs they lay are called nits. To find out if lice are thriving, look for nits; they are easier to see. Separate the hair in the area of the nape, and check for small white specks firmly attached to the base of the hair shaft. Another area to check is behind the ears. Once head lice or nits are found, immediately sanitize any combs or brushes used, and wash your hands, cape or towels that may have come in contact with the person's head. Also vacuum carpets and upholstery exposed to the person having pediculosis. Explain the situation in a confidential manner and indicate how to take care of this problem by using a specially medicated shampoo and following the doctor's instructions. The incidence of head lice infestation is on the rise and easily transmitted. Be on the lookout for signs of pediculosis. Intense itching on the back of the neck and head is one of the revealing symptoms of this condition. If any irritations are present in the scalp, question the person about these and determine if it will be safe to cut her hair.

Continue the analysis by selecting one strand of hair from the crown area; run your fingers down its length, stretching it. Repeat this same procedure with a strand taken from the nape area. If the strands do not break but show elasticity, by turning into a new curl when released, the hair is healthy and a trim can take care of the damaged ends. However, when half of the hair shafts turn into a new curl and brake easily, it means that the hair is structurally weak or severely damaged by chemicals. If only the strand selected from the crown shows damage, the person's activities or a careless styling routine are most likely drying and breaking her hair.

In the final step of hair analysis observe the following: Is the hair dry and rough? Are the ends split? Is the hair shaft faded or lacking shine? These observations may be done as you cut the hair, indicating in which areas you see damage. Find out about the person's activities, sports, hobbies, health, and hair care routine. For example: How does she style and take care of her hair? What kind of brush is she using? If she colors or waves her hair, how often is she doing it and what products and procedures is she using? How does she use the blow dryer? Does she use hot rollers? Does she protect her hair from the sun when she plays sports or goes to the beach? Is the hair brushed when wet rather than properly combed from the ends up? Is she on a diet? Are there any health and nutrition problems? The answers to these questions will give you clues to why the hair is damaged.

Hair that has been over-processed by a permanent wave or hair coloring will feel slippery when wet and mat easily. Unfortunately when hair has been treated with chemicals and over-processed it is virtually impossible to repair the damage. The best remedy is to gradually cut the damaged hair until new hair grows back. If the hair is coated with a metallic coloring agent it will look dull and lifeless. To protect hair from further damage, remove the metallic coating with a chemical remover, condition regularly and trim the damaged hair gradually.

As we mentioned in page 20, medium-textured hair and coarse hair have a tendency to feel dry. These two types of hair are especially sensitive to drying chemicals and to the environment in general. Low pH shampoos and conditioners will close the cuticle and give them shine. Remember that even when these types of hair are healthy and well-maintained, they will need special styling methods for a glamorous look.

Seasonal changes also affect the hair. During the winter months hair gets dry; whereas, in the summer, the oil glands are stimulated and the scalp and hair get oily. Since heating and air conditioning make hair dry and brittle, recommend changes in the type of shampoo and conditioner to compensate for sudden temperature changes, the harmful effects of the weather, outdoor sporting activities and other environmental conditions. Deep conditioning treatments will also help alleviate dry hair.

In the summer, it is a good idea to protect the hair from the harsh effects of the sun by selecting shampoos and conditioners that contain sunscreens. Most people these days no longer wear swim caps, but all types of hair need protection from salt and chlorinated or residue-laden water. For those who refuse to wear a swim cap, recommend a leave-in conditioner that will coat and protect the hair while swimming and that can be rinsed off afterwards. Clarifying gels--which help brake down salt, chlorine and chemical build-ups--can also be used while shampooing.

If the hair has been chemically processed, remind the person that her hair is particularly sensitive to dryness, fading, and uneven streaking. Suggest an easy care haircut and new looks with scarves and accessories that will keep the individual looking great.

Cleanliness is the most important step to beautiful hair. Some people don't wash their hair often enough, assuming that frequent shampooing will dry and damage their hair. This conception is incorrect. Even if the hair is dry, it should be washed frequently with special shampoo for dry hair and well conditioned for best results. Super-curly hair should be frequently washed to restore the moisture balance or it will be more prone to damage. Keratin conditioners, low ph shampoos conditioners, and deep conditioners are recommended for these types of hair. Emphasize that it is important to rinse thoroughly after shampooing and conditioning the hair.

Another point you need to discuss with the person is how the hair should be washed. Point out that stimulating the blood flow by massaging the scalp during each shampoo will maintain hair healthy. For this, the nails should not be used; they scratch and cause tears to the scalp making it sensitive and prone to infection and disease.

Brushing the hair from nape to top with the head down before retiring for the night is a timeless tip recommended to maintain healthy hair. Brushing increases the blood flow to the roots of the hair, keeps the scalp dandruff free, removes the daily dust from the hair and distributes the oils from the scalp to the dry ends. This procedure should be practiced regularly with a good brush that will not brake the hair or scratch the scalp. Make sure to analyze the hair before recommending this practice. If the hair lacks elasticity, brushing it in this fashion may cause breakage. If the hair is healthy, brushing it twenty to thirty times is sufficient.

Regular trims also help keep the hair healthy and beautiful. Trims eliminate old, faded hair and split ends. If split ends are not cut, they will keep splitting along the length of the hair until they brake off, leaving yet another split end behind to continue the process. If the person is trying to grow her hair long and refuses to get trims, point out that this can be achieved by cutting only where it is necessary and by trimming less than the hair growth during the period between trims.

The key to helping others improve their hair is communication. The individual with the damaged hair can provide you with enough information about the daily mistreatment of her hair; you, as the professional, have the answers to correct it.

Happy haircuts!

APPENDIX

RESOURCES

Beauty Associations provide the Cosmetologist with support and communication through workshops, conventions, seminars, trade shows, insurance programs, and many other benefits. Be sure to contact them for information on their membership dues and offers.

BEAUTY ASSOCIATIONS

Aestheticians International Association   1-800-888-0752
3606 Prescott Suite C
Dallas, Tx 75219
Contact: Ron Renee, Founder/Chairman

Allied Cosmetologists's Inc. of Illinois   (312) 721-3721
2602 East 87th Street
Chicago, IL 60617
Contact: Lena Sounder, Executive Director

American Beauty Association   (312) 644-6610
111 East Wacker Drive
Suite 600
Chicago, IL 60601
Contact: Paul Dystra, Director

American Health and Beauty Aids Institute   (312) 644-6610
111 East Wacker Drive
Suite 600
Chicago, IL 60601
Contact: Geri Duncan Jones, Executive Director

Beauty and Barber Supply Institute Inc.   (201) 808-7444
271 Route 46 F 209
Fairfield, NJ 07006
Contact: Fred Polk, Executive Director

Chicago Cosmetologists Association Inc.
111 East Wacker Drive
Suite 600
Chicago, IL 60601
Contact: Fred A. Piattoni, Executive Director

Florida Cosmetology Association, Inc.   (803) 289-3693
1311 N. Westshore Blvd.
Suite 114
Tampa, FL 33607

Hair International   (704) 552-6233
1318 Starbrook Drive
P.O. Box 240361
Charlotte, NC 28210
Contact: Rhonda Ewell, Office Manager

National Association of Accredited　　　　　(703) 845-1333
Cosmetology Schools
5201 Leesburg Pike, Suite 205
Falls Church, VA 22041
Contact: Dr. James P. Murphy, Executive Director

National Association of　　　　　(402) 474-4244
Barber/Styling Schools
304 South 11th Street
Lincoln, NE 68508
Contact: Alice Howard, Secretary

National Beauty Culturists' League, Inc.　　(202) 332-2695
25 Logan Circle N.W.
Washington, D.C. 20005
Contact: Cleolis Richardson, President

National Cosmetology Association　　　　1-800-527-1683
Executive Office
3510 Olive Street
St. Louis, MO 63103
Contact: George Bright

National Interstate Council of
State Boards of Cosmetology
P.O. Box 687
Pierre, SD 57501
Contact: Lois Wiskur, President

World International Nail &　　　　　(714) 779-9883
Beauty Association
1221 N. Lakeview
Anaheim, CA 92807
Contact: Jim George

CANADA

Allied Beauty Association　　　　　(416) 225-2359
Suite 1001
2 Sheppard Avenue East
Box 42
Willowdale Ontario M2N 5Y7
Contact: Rene Vincent

International Chain Salon Association
c/o Lagrange 5
4211 Cambridge Street
North Burnaby, BC V5C 1H1
Contact: Don Eamer, Executive Director

180

ENGLAND

**Hairdressing Manufacturers' And
Wholesalers' Association Limited**
Clare Cottage, Oakbank
Haywards Heath
West Sussex RH16 1RR
UK
Contact: Jeffrey Smith, Secretary

GERMANY

**Landesverband Des
Fachgrosshandles Mit Seifen
Kosmetika Friseurbedarf
Tolettartikel Und Kurzwaren Fur
Das Land Nordrhein-Westfalen**
Postfach 10 06 05
41-00 Duisburg 1
West Germany
Contact: Willi H. Decher

PUBLICATIONS

USA

AHBIA News
111 E. Wacker Dr.
Suite 600
Chicago IL 60601

Quarterly paper. Covers Black's issues in the Cosmetology industry, news, trends.

American Salon
7500 Old Oak Boulevard
Cleveland, Ohio 44130

Monthly. Salon news, hairstyles, products.

Modern Salon
400 Knightsbridge Pkwy
Lincolnshire, IL 60069

Monthly. News, articles, tips, products.

CANADA

Canadian Hairdresser
5200 Dixie Rd. Suite 204
Mississauga, Ont L4W 1E4

Text in English. Bi-monthly. Products. Salon deco. Competition announcements.

FRANCE

La Coiffeur de France
1-3 place de la Bourse
75008 Paris

Monthly. Text in French. News, products, styles. Has quarterly supplement with news and techniques.

La Coiffure De Paris
38 Rue Jean-Mermoz
75008 Paris

Monthly. Text in French. Hairstyling trends and products. Write to agent in the USA: Modern Salon A Vance Publication P.O. Box 400, Prairie View IL 60069

Mariages
38 Rue Jean-Mermoz
75008 Paris

Quarterly. Text in French. Wedding hairdressing techniques step-by-step.

Peluquerias
229 Rue Saint-Honoré
75001 Paris

Monthly. Text in French. Hairstyles and techniques.

HONG KONG

Hair International
15th Floor, Lockhart Centre
301-307A Lockhart Road

Text in Chinese and English. Quarterly. Features hair care, Avant-Garde trends, techniques, products.

ENGLAND

Hair
Oakfield House
Perrymount Road
Haywards Heath, West Sussex RH 16 3 DH

Quaterly. Hairstyle selection guide with 250 different styles.

Hairdressers Journal International
Quadrant House The Quadrant
Sutton Surrey SM2 5AS

Weekly. Hair design competition news. Interviews. Tips on hair color, hairstyles. Classified.

Recommended Productions

For information about the books and videotapes listed below, write to Good Life Products Inc., P.O. Box 170070, Hialeah, FL 33017-0070.

BOOKS

Finding and Keeping Clients- Audiocassette by Jane Segerstrom

Gran' Chic- 40 photographs of modern hairstyles for men and women and separate manual with techniques

Actiongroup Hairdesign- 38 photographs of modern hairstyles for men and women and separate manual with techniques

Coiffures de Paris- 30 new haircuts from Europe for women and children and separate manual with techniques

Style Trends- 36 haircuts for Black men and women and separate manual with techniques

Beautiful Braids and More Beautiful Braids- manual with step-by-step instructions to braid hair, 64 pages each manual

VIDEOTAPES

Les Vagabondes- Advanced haircutting By Tele-Coiffure showing how to cut Bob, Wedge and layered haircuts, VHS 60 minutes

Color Concepts- 30 advanced techniques to do bleaching, stripping, frosting streaking, blending and contrasting, VHS 90 minutes

Perm Concepts- Six perming techniques to produce volume on long and short hair, Asian and Ethnic hair, VHS 45 minutes

Styling Concepts- The latest advanced designs to create fabulous hairdos on all types of hair, VHS 45 minutes

Cutting Concepts- Shows how to cut short layers, style the hair and reduce bulk, VHS 62 minutes

Best of Clipper Cutting- Advanced clipper cutting, shows how to cut Bob, Wedge and layers VHS 30 minutes

Basic Clipper Techniques I- Step-by-step techniques to cut beard, moustache, men's hair, Bob, Wedge and modern Flattop, VHS 30 minutes

Basic Clipper Techniques II- Clipper cuts and lining for Black clients. Shows A-symmetrical weightline, ladies box cut, A-line cut, and Bi-level male design, VHS 30 minutes

Bibliography

Blanchard, Leslie. *Foolproof Guide to Beautiful Hair.* New York: Dalton, 1988.

Borston, Maurice and Bloomfield, Norma. *How to Blow Style.* Nottinhorn: Permaid Publications, 1975.

Chadwick, John. *The Chadwick System: Discovering the Perfect Hairstyle for You.* New York: Volkmann, 1982.

Charles, Ann. *The History of Hair.* New York: Bonanza, 1970.

Colletti, Anthony B. *Cosmetology The Keystone Guide to Beauty Culture.* Seventh Edition. New York. Keystone Publications, 1981.

Fodera, Sal. *Family Guide to Haircutting and Styling.* Drake, 1977.

Fine, Linda Sue. *The Complete Book of Hair Care, Hairstyling and Hairstylists.* New York: Arco Publishing, 1980.

Hofler, Robert. *Wild Style.* New York: Simon & Schuster, 1985.

*Home Haircutting Made Easy/*by the editors of Consumer Guide. New York: Bukman House: Distributed by Crown Publishers, 1980.

Jones, Jim. *Cutting & Comebacks.* Michigan: Jim Jones Enterprises, 1988.

Kenneth's Complete Book on Hair. Garden City. New York: Doubleday, 1972.

Layne, Lisa. *The Simple Guide to Home Haircutting.* New York: Pinnacle Books, 1982.

Michael, George. *George Michael's Secrets for Beautiful Hair.* George Michael and Lindsay. Garden City. New York: 1981.

Morrison, Maggie. *Glamour Guide to Hair.* New York: Fawcett Columbine, 1986.

Ohnstad, Bob. *Scissors and Comb Haircutting.* Minneapolis, Minn.: You can Publish, 1985.

Punches, Laurie. *How to Simply Cut Hair.* South Lake Tahoe, Ca.: Punches Productions, 1989.

Punches, Laurie. *How to Simply Cut Children's Hair.* South Lake Tahoe, Ca.: Punches Productions, 1989.

Punches, Laurie, *How to Simply Cut Hair Even Better.* South Lake Tahoe, Ca.: Punches Productions, 1989.

Roppatte, Vincent. *The Looks Men Love.* New York: St. Martin's Press, 1985.

Schoen, Linda Allen. *The Look You Like*: Paul Lazar. New York: M. Dekker, c 1990.

Taylor, Carolyn. *Carolyn's Taylor's Home Haircuts and Styles for Women and Girls.* Burley/Idaho. Anderson Publishing Co., 1988.

Taylor, Carolyn. *Carolyn's Taylor's Home Haircuts and Styles for Men and Boys.* Burley/Idaho. Anderson Publishing Co., 1989.

The AMA Book of Skin and Hair Care. ed. Linda Allen Schoen. Philadelphia and New York: J.B. Lippincott, 1986.

Glossary

attachments- comb that snaps over the blade of the clipper to provide a distace from the scalp

blunt cut- hair cut straight across

circulation- passage of blood through the body

coarse hair- hair fiber large in diameter

coif- hairstyle

concave- curved inward

conditioner- product that coats the hair to improve the appearance and feel of the hair

contract- shrink

convex- surface that curves outward, opposed to concave

cowlick- tuft of hair forming a spiral turn

degree- unit of measure for angles

density- thickness

dexterity- skill

diffuser- hair-blower attachment to spread the air and heat

Ducktail- style for the back of the head. The hair meets in the center

dry hair- hair devoid of enough natural oils

elasticity- capacity of the hair to stretch

elevate- lift

extend- stretch out

fine hair- term to identify the texture of the hair fiber small in diameter

graduations- lengths

hairline- edge of the scalp where the hair begins

horizontal- parallel to the ground. From left to right as opposed to up and down

increase- to become greater in size

limp- lacking firmness or strength

methodical- orderly, systematical

medium hair- term to identify the texture of the hair fiber between fine and coarse

nozzle- hair-blower attachment that directs the hair to one spot

pediculosis- headlice

perimeter- outer boundary

pH- the symbol for hydrogen ion concentration. pH scale expresses the degree of acidity or alkalinity in numbers from 0 to 14.

precision haircutting- haircut with exactness, where the lengths are measured and even

profile- side view of the face

progressive- successive steps

radial brush- round brush

scrunch drying- technique to curl the hair with the hand while blow-drying it

spikes- hair standing up

symmetrical- similar form on either side of the head

tapered- gradually decreasing hair length

texture- quality of the hair, coarse, medium or fine

vent brush- brush designed to allow the air pass through it and speed drying

vertical- perpendicular to the ground. Moving up and down as opposed to left and right

widow's peak- V shaped hairline at the middle of the forehead

INDEX

BOOK AND VIDEOCASSETTE PRODUCTIONS

The Haircoloring Manual
A practical guide to successful haircoloring
by Martha G. Fernandez

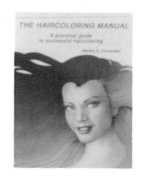

Here is the most comprehensive, practical, and up-to-date information available—information that will help you create the best haircolor for your client. This book is essential for every student, teacher and beauty salon's library; an effective haircoloring reference. Learn how to determine the right color for your client, how to correct haircolor mistakes, how to customize a formula, how to effectively apply haircolor, how to retouch, give highlights and decolorize hair. Contains more than 20 reference charts and a full color wheel indicating color depth, levels, tones, complementary colors to correct hair discoloration and more.

paper   0-944460-22-4 $18.95

Haircutting Basics
Revised and expanded edition
An easy, step-by-step guideto cutting hair the professional way

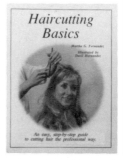
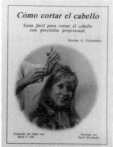

Noted teacher and hair artist, Martha Fernandez, introduces an innovative learning format and method to teach how to cut the most popular haircuts. Over 250 illustrations with instructions show each step of the techniques. Contains index, bibliography, glossary and resources guide.

paper   0-944460-21-6 $16.95
Spanish   0-944460-10-0 $16.95

Haircutting Basics VHS

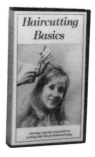
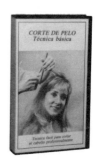

This excellent video shows the technique explained in the book. Teaches how to elevate the hair, establish and follow guides, how to cut short and long layers, the Bob and the Wedge haircuts. Fully narrated, live models.

ISBN   0-944460-13-5 VHS, Color, 45 min. $24.95
Spanish   0-944460-16-X

Braiding Beautiful VHS
Basic and Advanced Techniques

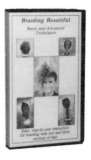
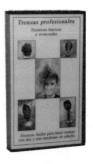

Renowned hair artist, Ines Yimoc, teaches how to create gorgeous braids for all occasions with two and three sections of hair, and how to adorn them for glamor. Step-by-step easy techniques to do the Fishtail, Cobra, Cornrow and the invisible French braids. Fully narrated, live models.

ISBN   0-944460-17-8 VHS, Color, 30 min. $19.95
Spanish   0-944460-18-6

Haircutting With Clippers VHS
Basic Techniques

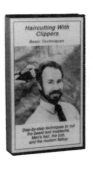
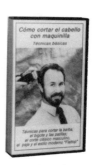

This videotape presents step-by-step techniques to cut and shape the beard, mustache and sideburns; men's hair, the Bob and the modern Flattop. A complete clipper cutting course for the beginner with the latest techniques. Fully narrated, live models.

ISBN   0-944460-19-4 VHS, Color, 30 min. $19.95
Spanish   0-944460-20-8

Write to us for Free brochure with additional products

ORDER FORM

		Quantity	Total
The Haircoloring Manual (book)	@ $18.95	_____	_____
Haircutting Basics (book)	@ $16.95	_____	_____
Haircutting Basics (videotape)	@ $24.95	_____	_____
Braiding Beautiful (videotape)	@ $19.95	_____	_____
Haircutting With Clippers (videotape)	@ $19.95	_____	_____
SPANISH TITLES			
Cómo cortar el cabello (libro)	@ $16.95	_____	_____
Corte de pelo - técnica básica (video)	@ $24.95	_____	_____
Trenzas profesionales (video)	@ $19.95	_____	_____
Cómo cortar el cabello con maquinilla (video)	@ $19.95	_____	_____

Shipping: $2.00 for the first item and $0.50 for each additional item _____

Total _____

Name _____ Phone (____) _____

Address _____

City/State/Zip _____

We only accept **American Express**

Acct. # [| | | | | | | | | | | | | |]

____ My check/Money Order is enclosed
____ Bill my American Express Card

_____ Expires: ____
Signature

Mail to: *Beauty Ed*, P. O. Box 170070, Hialeah, FL 33017-0070

ORDER FORM

		Quantity	Total
The Haircoloring Manual (book)	@ $18.95	_____	_____
Haircutting Basics (book)	@ $16.95	_____	_____
Haircutting Basics (videotape)	@ $24.95	_____	_____
Braiding Beautiful (videotape)	@ $19.95	_____	_____
Haircutting With Clippers (videotape)	@ $19.95	_____	_____
SPANISH TITLES			
Cómo cortar el cabello (libro)	@ $16.95	_____	_____
Corte de pelo - técnica básica (video)	@ $24.95	_____	_____
Trenzas profesionales (video)	@ $19.95	_____	_____
Cómo cortar el cabello con maquinilla (video)	@ $19.95	_____	_____

Shipping: $2.00 for the first item and $0.50 for each additional item _____

Total _____

Name _____ Phone (____) _____

Address _____

City/State/Zip _____

We only accept **American Express**

Acct. # [| | | | | | | | | | | | | |]

____ My check/Money Order is enclosed
____ Bill my American Express Card

_____ Expires: ____
Signature

Mail to: *Beauty Ed*, P. O. Box 170070, Hialeah, FL 33017-0070

ABOUT THE AUTHOR

In 1968, at age fourteen, Martha Fernandez fled Cuba with her parents to seek political refuge in Spain. Two years later, she came to the United States where she resumed her education at El Monte High School in California.

In 1973, she moved to Miami where she attended Florida International University and graduated in Education. Years later she obtained a cosmetologist license and with her text, *Haircutting Basics,* published for the first time in 1986, she has become a leading writer and educator in the field of Cosmetology. Her book has been acclaimed by teachers and students of Cosmetology all over the nation and has been used in over 2,000 schools of Cosmetology.

She has settled in Miami with her husband and three children and has promised, after all her tribulations, to never move again.